PILATES
for pregnancy

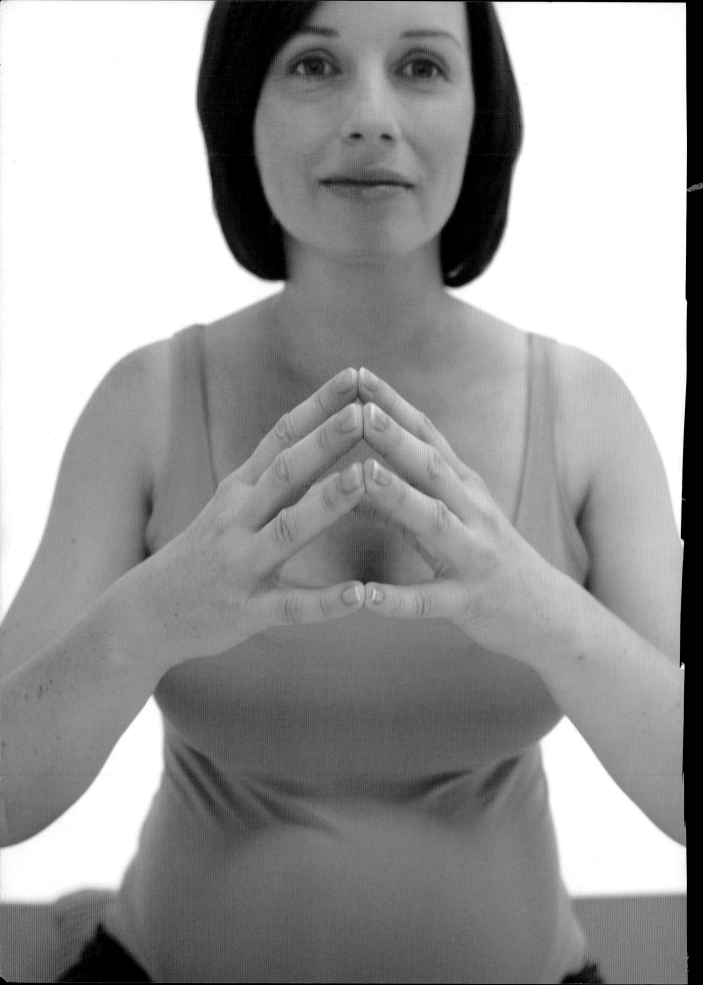

hamlyn

PILATES
for pregnancy

Safe and natural exercises for before and after the birth

JAN ENDACOTT

Jan Endacott enjoyed a successful
career as a professional dancer before
becoming a personal trainer specializing
in women's fitness. Jan, a mother of two
children, is a qualified Pilates instructor,
fitness trainer and sports psychologist.
Her exercise programmes have helped
women to achieve their personal fitness
goals before, during and after pregnancy.
She is the author of *The Fitball Workout*.

First published in Great Britain in 2007
by Hamlyn, a division of
Octopus Publishing Group Ltd
2–4 Heron Quays, London E14 4JP

Distributed in the United States and Canada by
Sterling Publishing Co., Inc.
387 Park Avenue South, New York, NY 10016-8810

10 9 8 7 6 5 4 3 2 1

Printed and bound in China

ISBN-13: 978-0-600-61580-4
ISBN-10: 0-600-61580-4

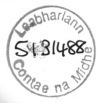

SAFETY NOTE
It is advisable to check with your doctor first before
embarking on any exercise programme. Pilates should
not be regarded as a replacement for professional medical
treatment, a physician should be consulted in all matters
relating to health and particularly in respect of pregnancy
and any symptoms which may require diagnosis or
medical attention. While the advice and information in this
book is believed to be accurate and the instructions given
have been devised to avoid strain, neither the author nor
the publisher can accept any legal responsibility for any
injury sustained while following the exercises.

CONTENTS

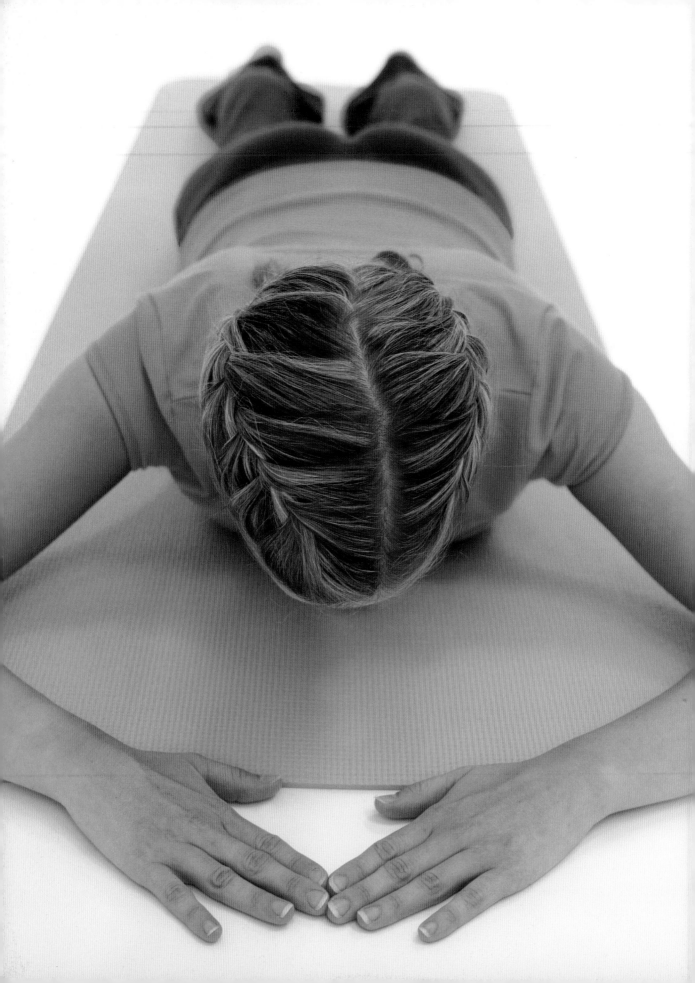

INTRODUCTION

Congratulations on reading this book! It means two exciting things. First, that you are pregnant; and second, that you want to be fit and healthy before and after the birth of your baby. The gentle approach of Pilates makes it an ideal choice of exercise throughout pregnancy, which will help you to improve and maintain your levels of fitness without strain.

Pregnancy is a fascinating time when your body's shape and needs change constantly as your pregnancy progresses. These changes create new and different demands on your muscles and joints, so it is essential that your exercise routine adapts to accommodate these new challenges.

Pilates is the ideal form of exercise to make your pregnancy and the birth more comfortable, with its focus on core stability, the pelvic floor and gently strengthening and toning the muscles. It enhances concentration and enables you to develop a unique relationship with your body when you exercise — especially important during pregnancy. Pilates not only helps to improve your central strength, but also your balance, your coordination and the quality of your movement, without placing stress on your joints.

With its emphasis on developing good posture, which can easily nose-dive during pregnancy, Pilates will help to prevent backache, slumped shoulders and neck tension. Your pregnancy is the perfect opportunity to make life-enhancing changes, and this book will assist you in making the most of this very special time.

BENEFITS OF PILATES DURING PREGNANCY

- Pilates is an extremely safe and effective method of exercising during pregnancy. By focusing on the postural muscles you will improve your core stability and pelvic-floor strength, which will help you stand tall and avoid backache.

- Practising Pilates during pregnancy gives you great abdominal tone. Stronger abdominals provide better support and enable your spine to lengthen. The resulting improvement in your posture gives your baby more room.

- Pilates is respected and recommended by the medical profession. The specially adapted toning and strengthening exercises help to alleviate the aches and pains often associated with the changes that are taking place in your body.

- Pilates improves circulation. All movements are initiated from your abdominal muscles, improving circulation in the abdomen, which is beneficial for your baby.

- The increased relaxation and calming effects derived from Pilates exercises during pregnancy may transfer some unique health benefits to your growing baby.

- With its carefully controlled approach, Pilates enables you to develop increased body awareness. You will learn to relax and breathe correctly in preparation for labour and your baby's birth.

- Practising Pilates exercises regularly during and after pregnancy promotes good recovery from labour and the birth, giving you the basis to regain your former figure with the post-natal programme.

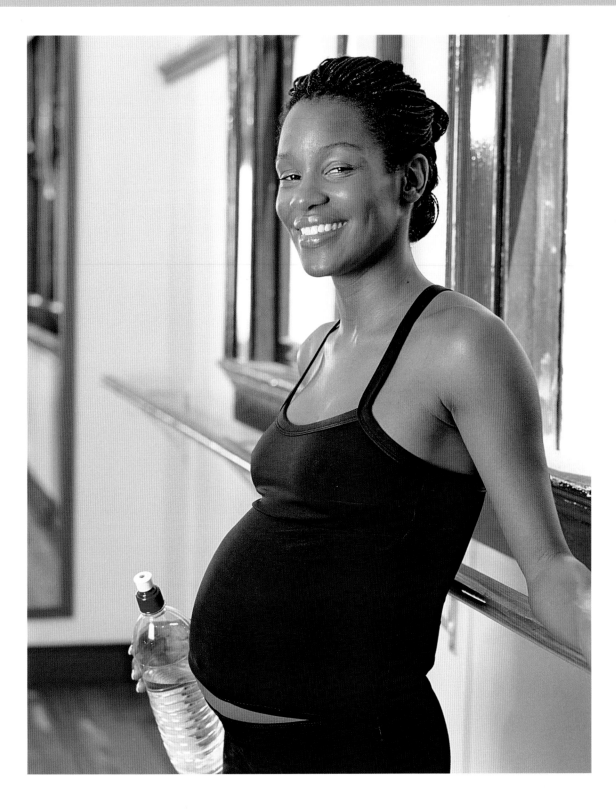

YOUR CHANGING BODY

Nothing quite prepares you for the number of amazing changes that your body undergoes in such a short space of time. Every woman experiences pregnancy in a uniquely different way, but the changes that occur during these nine months are set off by floods of hormones. Understanding the changes that are happening will help you to feel more at ease.

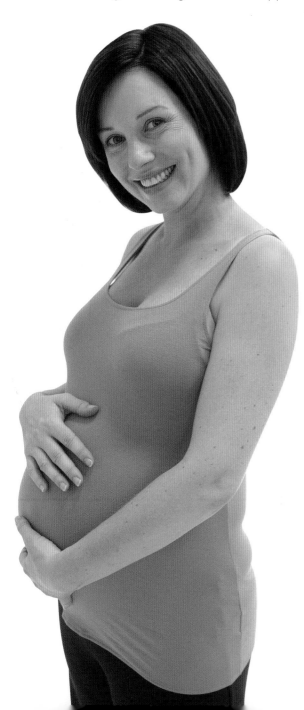

HORMONES

The hormones mainly responsible for creating the perfect conditions for pregnancy and your growing baby are oestrogen and progesterone. Levels of these hormones increase dramatically, and your muscles yield to provide the ideal environment for your baby.

Another hormone that increases is relaxin, which causes the ligaments that provide joint stability to become more supple. The joints that hold the bones of the pelvis together gradually loosen, preparing you for labour and the birth. However, joint stability is weakened. It is therefore vital that good alignment and correct posture are maintained. Pilates encourages core muscle control, which compensates for the weakened ligaments, helping you to avoid common joint problems and back strain.

Other hormones that increase are the positive mood-enhancing ones known as endorphins. These not only increase your own feelings of well being, but pass their positive effects across the placenta to your baby. If you feel at all anxious or stressed during pregnancy, Pilates also teaches you to relax and breathe efficiently, inducing calm and effectively reducing levels of the stress hormone cortisol, which may rise at this time (see 'Breathing Technique' and 'Relaxation' on pages 28 and 30).

INCREASED BLOOD VOLUME

Your growing body needs to produce more blood, and by full term your blood volume increases by 30–40 per cent and your heart has to work much harder to pump all that blood around your body. The Pilates exercises in this book will not over-raise your heart rate, for over-exertion may cause dizzy spells. Your baby's heart rate is already faster than yours, so it is vital not to over-accelerate your own.

CIRCULATION

Hormonal changes may also affect the valves in your veins that normally prevent the back-flow of blood. This may sometimes lead to varicose veins and/or haemorrhoids, and your increased weight gain and raised blood volume exacerbate this. Pilates movements help to boost circulation in the lower limbs.

FLUID RETENTION

Levels of lymphatic fluid, amniotic fluid and fluid to all tissues in the body increase during pregnancy. Regular exercise helps to prevent fluid build-up from causing conditions such as water retention and swelling (oedema). Feeling tired, headaches, lethargy and poor concentration are often caused by a lack of water. It is therefore essential to drink at least eight glasses of water each day, and up to 12 if you're exercising, in order to ensure you keep well hydrated.

DIGESTIVE SYSTEM

An early, unpleasant symptom of pregnancy is nausea or vomiting, which usually lessens or stops by mid-pregnancy. To reduce nausea, avoid letting your stomach get too empty. Eat small amounts more frequently, avoid eating heavy meals close to bedtime, and keep up your fluid intake to avoid dehydration. During pregnancy your digestive process slows down, which often causes heartburn, indigestion or constipation. A balanced diet rich in fresh, unrefined and unprocessed foods will keep you and your baby in optimum health.

BREAST-SIZE INCREASE

In early pregnancy your breast size increases. Heavier breasts add stress to your upper body, causing your shoulders to slump forwards and creating a stooped posture. Pilates exercises will reduce tension in the upper back and shoulders and enhance postural awareness.

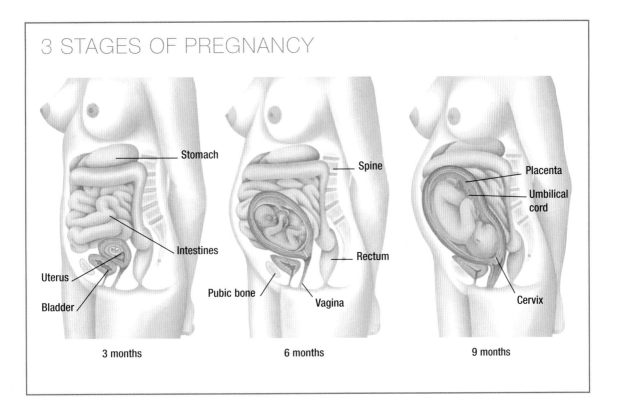

3 STAGES OF PREGNANCY

3 months

6 months

9 months

A well-fitting bra will provide essential support and comfort; you may need several fittings throughout your pregnancy and when breastfeeding.

ABDOMINAL MUSCLE SEPARATION: DIASTASIS RECTI

As your baby grows, your uterus expands and your stomach muscles stretch. The rectus abdominis muscles (known as 'the six-pack') stretch and separate to allow for this expansion. This separation is called 'diastasis recti' and is experienced by about two-thirds of pregnant women. If you experience this separation of the rectus abdominis muscles, you should not perform any traditional curl-up exercises, because you no longer have sufficient support. We often think of the six-pack as the muscles to train to flatten our tummies. However, Pilates will show you how to exercise your central core muscles so that you can safely recover your waistline.

CENTRAL SUPPORT MUSCLES

Pilates focuses on the centre of your torso, the postural muscles at your body's core. This centre is made up of the abdominal muscles, the back and the buttocks. Pilates exercises initiate all movements from this central core. One of the most important muscles is the deep-seated abdominal muscle called the transversus abdominis. It emerges from your pelvis into your ribcage and diaphragm, wrapping itself around your middle like a corset or wide belt. This muscle helps to support your baby as well as your spine. A strong transversus muscle will help to stop your pelvis tilting too far forwards, which can cause lower-spine discomfort during the last stages of pregnancy. It is also the main muscle used during labour and, because you 'push' with it, you need to strengthen it to cope with all these demands.

SEPARATION OF THE PUBIS SYMPHYSIS

The pubis symphysis joins the pubic bones together at the front of the pelvis, forming a cushion of cartilage that plays a major role in helping to provide stability in the pelvis. In preparation for birth, your pelvis changes shape as the hormone relaxin enables the joint to loosen and separate, facilitating the expansion needed for your baby to pass through at birth. You should avoid any activities that cause you to experience pain in this area.

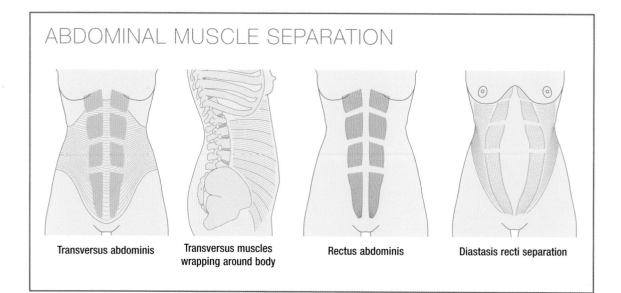

ABDOMINAL MUSCLE SEPARATION

Transversus abdominis

Transversus muscles wrapping around body

Rectus abdominis

Diastasis recti separation

PELVIC FLOOR

Pilates exercises focus on core strength and stabilization. Your pelvic floor forms an integral part of that core, helping to support the growing uterus, and must remain strong and elastic to cope with the demands of pregnancy and labour. The pelvic-floor muscles act like a hammock, passing from the pubic bone at the front of your pelvis to the coccyx at the back and out to each side of the ischium – your 'sit-bones', which you can locate by sitting on a firm chair, placing your hands under your buttocks and feeling for the bony protuberances as you rock from side to side. The urethra, vagina and anus separate this hammock-like band of muscle.

Surrounding the urethra, vagina and anus is a figure of eight muscle called the pubococcygeus. Strengthening the pubococcygeus will help to alleviate or prevent potential bowel or bladder problems which can be particularly troublesome during pregnancy. Strong pelvic-floor muscles hold your internal organs in place, help stop embarrassing urinary leaks, and assist during labour. Toned muscles are not only strong, but, surprisingly, are also more elastic and therefore will stretch with ease when the hormone relaxin kicks in to enable the pelvic

floor muscles to stretch and relax during childbirth. This combination helps make labour and birth a more comfortable experience. Strong pelvic-floor muscles have multiple benfits, which are important for your health even when you are not pregnant.

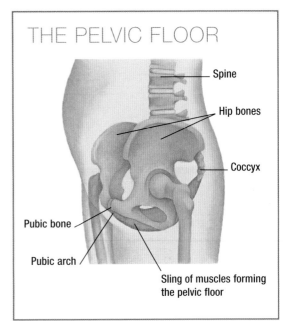

THE PELVIC FLOOR

- Spine
- Hip bones
- Coccyx
- Pubic bone
- Pubic arch
- Sling of muscles forming the pelvic floor

BENEFITS OF A STRONG PELVIC FLOOR

- Improves the ability to stretch and relax more easily during childbirth.

- Improves circulation to the pelvic region.

- Promotes fast recovery and healing, helping to regain muscle tone after birth.

- Prevents stress incontinence.

- Improves sexual sensations.

- Supports the pelvic organs.

- Prevents poor alignment of the hip and sacro-iliac joints (which form an interface between the back of the pelvis and the hip bones).

- Helps prevent bowel and bladder problems which may occur in later life.

- Promotes core stability.

For ways to strengthen the pelvic floor, follow the pelvic exercises on pages 32–33.

TAKING CARE OF YOUR POSTURE

One of the first things you notice as your pregnancy develops is your posture changing, which causes many women to experience back pain. This chapter will provide you with essential awareness skills and techniques which are designed to enhance your posture and protect your spine during a variety of everyday activities.

Correct posture is vital to protect your spine before, during and after your pregnancy. During pregnancy the growing weight, size and load you are carrying on the front of your body all contribute to placing stress on your lower back. This can cause you to compensate by adopting a poor posture in your upper spine. As your balance alters, your centre of gravity shifts (see diagram below). Pilates will enable you to identify the key muscles that are essential in creating correct posture and will teach you how to use those muscles without tension or forced movements. You will be rewarded with a balanced body that will project poise, grace and ease of movement.

POSTURE

During pregnancy you will be putting on a considerable amount of weight – possibly up to 14 kg (30 lb) – the bulk of which will be carried on the front of your body. Your heavier breasts will impose a forward pull on your shoulders which will cause slouching, while your growing abdomen will move your centre of balance forwards and upwards. The normal curvature of your spine will become exaggerated, hollowing your back and instigating lower back pain. Control and stability are therefore required from your central core muscles. Good posture has lifetime benefits and makes you look and feel confident while protecting against pains and strains. Check your own posture by standing sideways in front of a long mirror.

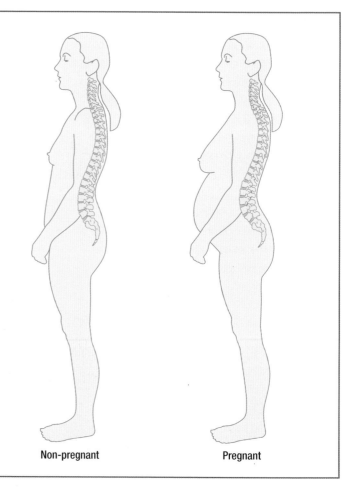

Non-pregnant   Pregnant

SELF-AWARENESS

How we feel emotionally has a direct bearing on how we hold ourselves. Visualize how someone appears when they lack confidence: you will probably conjure up a picture of a bowed head, lowered eye-line and stooped shoulders. Your vision of someone who is over-confident or arrogant will probably have a raised chin and squared shoulders. A miserably tired person may have a stooped neck, rounded shoulders and will appear slumped. These examples demonstrate how posture offers a reflection of our innermost feelings, providing an advertisement to the world of our disposition and personality.

The following pages will help you become instinctively aware of your posture and the body language that you project. This may involve changing many of the bad postural habits that you have adopted without realizing it. Bad practices – such as slouching, sitting into one hip, rounding your shoulders, walking, standing, bending and carrying incorrectly – can all be corrected by retraining your muscle memory. This will instil in you an automatic and instinctive self-awareness.

Ballet dancers are perfect examples of people who have automatic self-awareness. They appear to possess a natural grace when they stand and walk, and even when they do the shopping! This is because their movements and actions are slowly rehearsed and practised methodically until they become second nature. Their muscle memory becomes programmed to move instinctively with good posture, grace and ease.

Pilates movements follow the same principles of controlled, mindful exercise that dancers use. They will help you gain self-awareness by guiding you through easy-to-follow, structured movement patterns, which focus on posture and correct body alignment that will flow into your everyday movements and activities. Better posture will help to prevent backache and joint stress in pregnancy. It will also make you feel more confident and positive, increase your vitality and boost your energy levels.

STANDING WITH GOOD POSTURE

To achieve good posture in pregnancy, you need to do the following:

- Stand with your feet hip-width apart, with your weight evenly distributed between your big toes, little toes and heels (visualize a tripod).

- Relax your knees.

- Avoid gripping your buttocks.

- Ensure that your pelvis is in neutral alignment (this means not over-tilting it forwards or backwards); drop your tailbone towards the floor.

- Hang your arms loosely at your sides and relax your ribs; feel a sense of width across your shoulder blades and of breadth across your chest.

- Release any tension from your neck, and relax and soften your jaw muscles; imagine a piece of string attached to the top of your head pulling you up towards the ceiling.

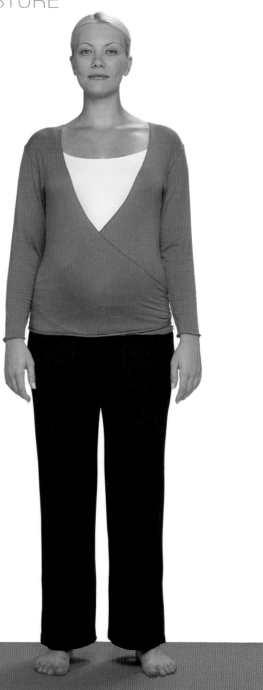

WALKING WITH POISE

Walking is the most natural form of movement and will increase the circulation to your legs. Follow these guidelines for good posture:

- Wear comfortable footwear and roll through your feet as you walk; avoid wearing high heels, as they will throw your posture off-centre.

- As you walk, swing your arms gently without tensing your hands, neck or shoulders.

- If standing for long periods is unavoidable, move your feet by scrunching your toes, then rise up on tiptoes or walk on the spot to keep your circulation stimulated and to avoid potential cramp.

SITTING WITH GOOD POSTURE

When you sit with good posture, your spine adopts a shallow S-shape. After sitting for some time, your posture sags and you will end up with a 'banana-shaped' back. Unfortunately soft, deep chairs encourage your spine into this bad habit. To maintain a good sitting posture you must:

- Make sure your back is supported – if necessary, use a small cushion or rolled-up towel in the small of your back to support your lower spine.

- Place your feet flat on the floor.

- Pull up tall from the top of your head, keeping your spine in the S-shape and relaxing your shoulders to avoid tension.

- Avoid crossing your legs, and keep the backs of your knees slightly away from the seat to prevent poor circulation.

- Ensure that your chair has adjustable height and angle if you are in a working environment; when using a computer, your chair-to-desk height is correct if your wrists and forearms are parallel or sloping down to the work surface.

STANDING FROM A SEATED POSITION

- Ensure that your feet are hip-width apart, with one foot slightly in front of the other.

- Lean forwards over your thighs and stand up using the strength of your legs, not your back.

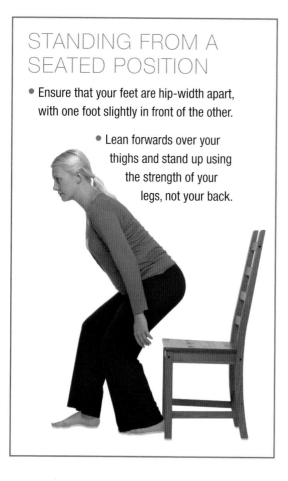

BENDING AND CARRYING SAFELY

- When you need to lift something up from floor level, bend down to it using your knees, keeping your back as straight as you can.

- Keep the load as close to your torso as possible, and use your strong leg muscles to do the work by straightening your legs.

- Hold the load in both hands; if it is too heavy, get someone else to do it!

- When carrying shopping bags, distribute the weight evenly between both hands to aid balance and avoid strain.

- All jobs around the home and garden at floor level are easier to do by sitting at the level of the task in hand – on the floor; this avoids unnecessary bending for prolonged periods.

SITTING UPRIGHT FROM LYING DOWN

You must always take care not to strain your spine as you sit up from lying down, particularly in the later stages of pregnancy when there is more pressure on your abdominal muscles. Avoid any sudden movements when sitting up. Pilates exercises will help you to develop smooth movement control. Bean bags and support cushions are great for relaxing on, because they help to alleviate lower back pain and neck ache. You can also use this technique when getting up from a lying-down exercise position.

- From lying down, roll onto one side and prop yourself up on one elbow.

- Keeping your knees and ankles together, swing your legs down off the side of the bed and bring your body up carefully into a sitting position in one smooth, controlled movement.

- Use your arms to help push you up from the sideways position.

SAFE LYING AND STANDING SEQUENCE

This four-step routine will help you get down and up from the floor safely. As your baby's weight increases, you may find your balance affected, so move more slowly and deliberately. Use this sequence from mid-pregnancy onwards, and continue until after your six-week post-natal check. This will help to speed your recovery after the birth.

- Pull your navel in towards your spine. Bend your knees and lower your body weight onto one knee, then transfer on to both knees.

- Keeping your navel pulled in towards your spine, put your hands on the floor in front of you. Now sit to one side and draw your knees up slightly.

- Using your elbows for support, slowly lower yourself back towards the floor. Move smoothly down in a controlled movement onto your back.

- To get up again, roll onto your side, bend your knees up and use your hands to push up into a side-sitting position. Turn onto your hands and knees, then come up onto one knee. Rest both hands on your front thigh and push up to stand upright.

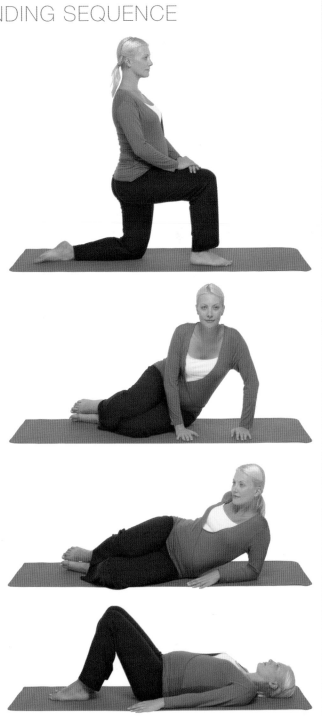

SAFE PRACTICE

You have wisely chosen Pilates to help you make every possible effort to ensure your body provides a healthy and calm environment in which your baby can be nurtured and grow. By following the exercise instructions and safety guidelines you will derive maximum benefit from the gentle nature of Pilates during this special time leading up to the baby's arrival.

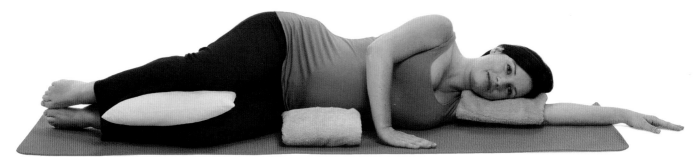

NEWCOMERS TO PILATES

Joseph Pilates, born in Germany in 1880, originally created his system of exercise to help him deal with his own physical problems brought about by childhood illness. He moved to England in 1912 and it was during the war years that he went on to develop his 'muscle contrology' system and his renowned mat-work exercises. His philosophy was to coordinate the mind, spirit and body to work *with* the body's muscles, not 'on' them.

CAUTION

- If you have not practised Pilates prior to pregnancy, it is advisable to postpone starting this programme until after your fourth month has passed, when your pregnancy should be secure.

- It is essential to exercise gently and carefully in early pregnancy, when the risk of miscarriage is at its peak.

If you are a newcomer to Pilates, you are about to embark on a system of exercise that will enhance your posture, fitness, health and general well being. The calm, controlled, flowing exercise movements provide the ideal exercise system for your pregnancy and for regaining your figure after the birth.

As a newcomer, you should commence Pilates after the fourth month of your pregnancy. Ensure that you learn the basic principles and follow most of the Early Pregnancy Workout — in other words, start at the beginning! Omit any exercises that require you to lie on your front, and do not perform any exercise lying on your back for longer than three minutes. Read the 'General training guidelines' (see pages 22–23) to ensure that you get the most from your Pilates workouts.

SAFETY DURING PREGNANCY

Generally women are encouraged to continue with their normal exercise routine during pregnancy, but not to exceed their pre-pregnancy intensity levels. However, it is a sensible precaution to check with your doctor for any special instructions. Every woman is unique, which means that you will need to constantly adapt and modify your exercise routine to allow for the many hormonal and physical changes that will occur during your pregnancy.

It is right to take every possible safety precaution, but pregnancy is not an illness! Have regular ante-natal checks to detect any medical changes, and you will then enjoy the benefits of gentle exercise throughout pregnancy and be well prepared for labour, childbirth and being a mum.

If you are suffering from any medical conditions, or problems or complications associated with your pregnancy, you must check with your doctor before embarking on any type of exercise programme. If you find that you start to experience any pain or discomfort or unusual symptoms during exercise, stop immediately and seek medical advice.

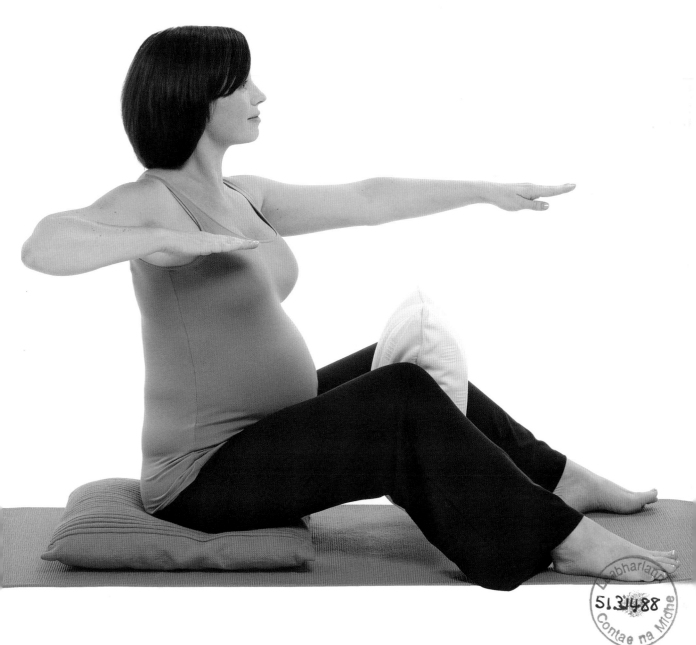

GENERAL TRAINING GUIDELINES

Wear loose, comfortable clothing that does not restrict your movement. Be particularly careful not to overheat during the first three months of pregnancy. Wear a good supportive bra that has been properly fitted, to help avoid stretch marks. Pilates is best practised without shoes; if you want to wear socks, make sure they have anti-slip soles.

EQUIPMENT

You will need the following small selection of equipment to enable you to get the best out of your Pilates programme:

- A thick padded exercise mat

- A sturdy chair with no arms

- A small flat pillow or folded towel, plus several plump cushions or pillows

- A yoga block

- A long scarf and an exercise band or stretchband

- A sponge ball and a softball

- A pair of light dumb-bells: about 0.45 kg (1lb) or 0.9 kg (2 lb) each weight

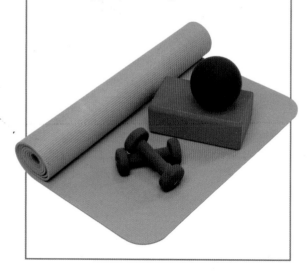

CHOOSING THE RIGHT EXERCISES

Selected exercises have been carefully chosen for each stage of pregnancy. Advice and specific guidelines for the various stages are given at the start of each section. Read the 'Safe practice' advice (see pages 20–21) before starting, and if you have an existing back complaint, seek your doctor's advice before commencing exercise.

WHEN TO EXERCISE

Late afternoon or early evening is physically the best time to exercise, when your muscles are warmed from the day's activities. However, your lifestyle may not permit this, because you are still working, have children to care for or perhaps are just a 'morning person'. It does take longer to warm up first thing in the day, but the most important thing is to find a time that is right for you. Whatever time you choose, develop a routine, stick to it and don't permit interruptions. Treat it as much a part of your life as cleaning your teeth after breakfast. Aim to achieve a balance between your exercising and family/work demands to ensure that you achieve a calm and relaxed mind and body. Keep a diary to chart your progress and help you stay on track.

WHERE TO EXERCISE

Choose a room with enough space to move around freely without restrictions or obstructions. Ideally, it should be quiet, not stuffy and at a comfortable temperature, with plenty of light. Make sure there are no chilly draughts. It is a good idea to keep your exercise equipment in the same room that you use for your workouts, as having to search out and carry it all from room to room may blunt your enthusiasm! Try to eliminate distractions (switch on your

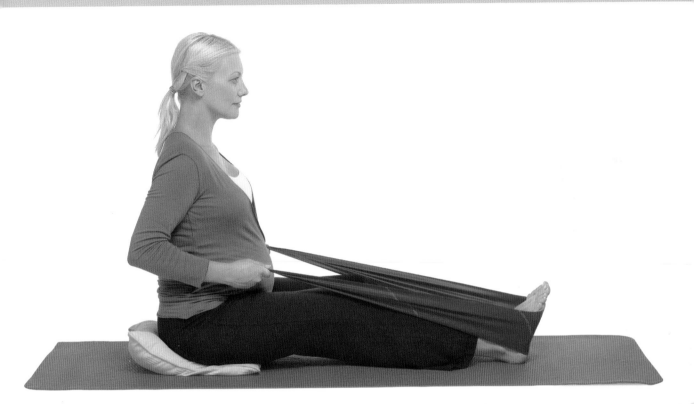

answer-phone) and create a comfortable atmosphere. Use background music if it helps; listening to music that you enjoy while you exercise can promote positive thoughts and feelings, which will help you feel more motivated and will achieve better results.

CARDIOVASCULAR EXERCISE

You need to complement your Pilates exercises with some moderate cardiovascular activity every day in order to balance your health and fitness objectives. If you have not been actively exercising before your pregnancy, you need to start aerobic exercise slowly and build up gradually. The safest types of cardiovascular exercise are walking and swimming.

Avoid any activities that put you and your baby at risk. Particularly hazardous are contact sports, deep-sea or scuba diving, hang-gliding, skydiving, water or downhill skiing, horse riding, ice skating, gymnastics, cycling, or any activity that may cause loss of balance.

NUTRITION

A well-balanced, healthy diet during pregnancy will provide optimum health for you and your baby. Eat fresh organic foods with plenty of fresh fruit and vegetables, wholegrain cereals, dairy products and protein foods. As far as possible, avoid processed and refined foods to help you cut out hidden salts, bad fats and chemically treated foods. Check with your midwife which foods are best avoided during pregnancy. If you suffer from morning sickness (which can occur at any time of day), keep dry crackers close to hand to help avert hunger, as this may be a pre-cursor to nausea. Food hygiene is also extremely important at this time. Drinking alcohol should be avoided during your pregnancy.

You should eat at regular times and never skip meals. It is better to eat smaller meals at frequent intervals each day than to have fewer, heavier meals. Consult a qualified dietary practitioner if you are vegetarian or vegan, or have any dietary allergies.

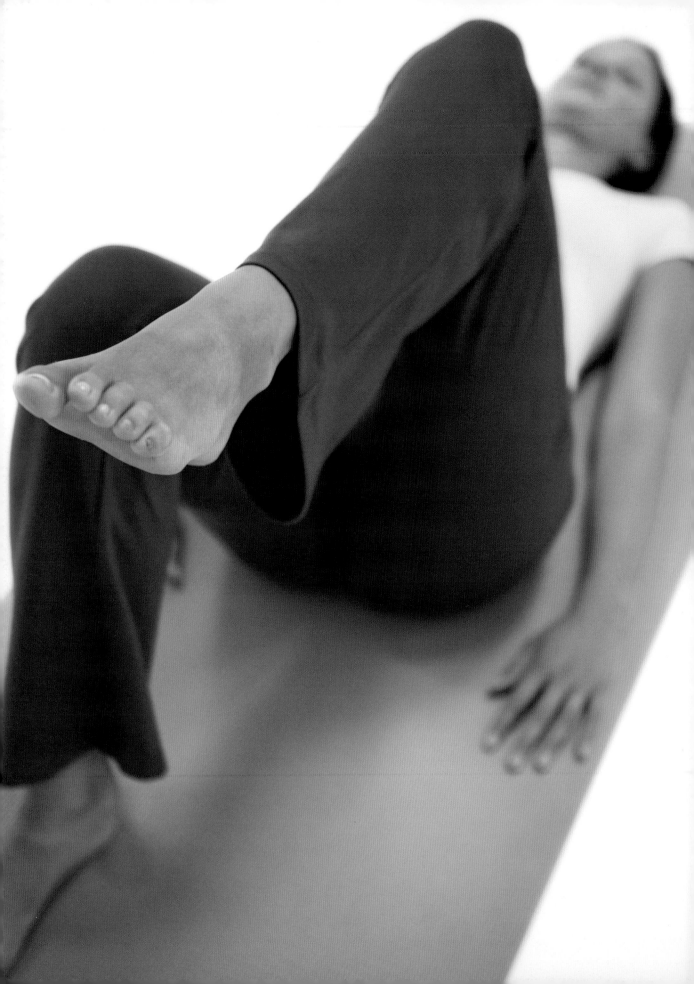

PILATES
BASICS

PILATES PRINCIPLES

There are different variations and interpretations of Joseph Pilates's system of exercise, but all are based on the following principles, which he established as being essential to acquiring optimum physical health.

Breathing efficiently is vital to your health and is one of the most important principles of Pilates. Learning how to breathe correctly will ensure that you derive maximum benefit from all the exercises.

The use of relaxation techniques encourages tranquillity and a calm, focused mind. This aids the concentration that Pilates requires, ensuring precise focus on the area of the body that is being exercised. Visualization is one of the most effective methods in Pilates of using the power of the mind to affect physical performance and results.

Core stability is the very foundation on which Pilates movements are based. The core muscles are the body's centre of strength, and provide the powerhouse from which all Pilates movements are initiated. The correct use of pelvic placement is designed to achieve a natural, neutral position for the spine and pelvis, helping to reduce stress on the spine. Shoulder stability exercises stabilize the shoulder blades and target the muscles that create better head and neck alignment. Correct head and neck placement is the top rung on the ladder of good posture.

BREATHING

Breathing correctly allows oxygen to enrich the blood and nourish the whole body. Shallow breathing, using just the upper part of the lungs, means that working muscles are starved of the oxygen they require. When you breathe in fully, oxygen-rich blood recharges the working muscles; and as you breathe out deeply, your body releases non-beneficial waste and chemicals from your blood. Pilates exercises encourage breathing deeply into the lower lobes of the lungs to help this exchange process. Practising proper breathing will help you to avoid tension and enable you to focus on maintaining correct exercise movements.

RELAXATION

Pilates is a wonderful way to work out gently in pregnancy without creating undue tension in your body. It may seem strange to suggest that a fitness workout can be described as relaxing, but this is exactly what Pilates sets out to be. Pilates provides exercises that initiate from a relaxed, calm start position and are designed to challenge your body, using flowing, controlled movements in a smooth, precise way. This relaxed approach to gaining and maintaining fitness benefits your baby as well!

CONCENTRATION

We all suffer from internal 'chitter-chatter'– that constant background nagging about all the outstanding tasks of the day: 'get the shopping', 'remember sister's birthday card', and so on. To gain the most from your Pilates exercises it is vital to develop the ability to cut out this mental background noise and concentrate your thoughts and energy on the area of the body that you are exercising. This enables you to target your exercise specifically to produce the maximum result. A calm, focused start and finish to your Pilates workouts are especially beneficial when you are pregnant.

VISUALIZATION

During pregnancy you become more in tune with your body and will naturally develop a heightened sense of self-awareness. Visualization helps to harness this into a technique that sportspeople in particular use to improve performance and results. It is particularly useful during relaxation, when it enables you to use your mind and imagination to enhance your exercise technique. Your new-found inner calm will help you feel in control of your changing body.

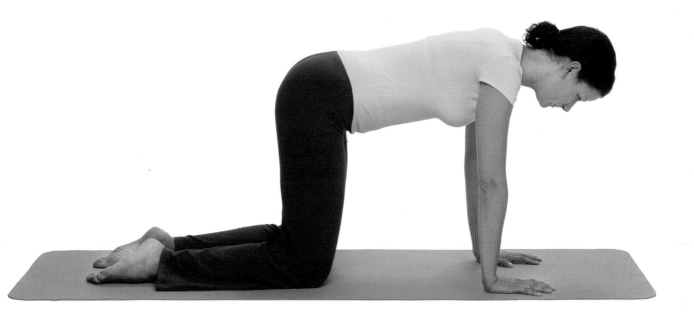

CORE STABILITY

The central core is known as the powerhouse of the body from which all Pilates movements and strength emanate. A strong central core provides a muscular framework that supports your posture, spine and pelvis. Developing and maintaining strong core muscles throughout your pregnancy will help to avoid the back pain many women suffer, caused by the shift in the body's centre of gravity as it moves upwards and forwards, distorting the natural curve of the spine. During pregnancy, core stability helps your body to rebalance as your baby grows larger and to alleviate the additional stresses and strains on your joints. In the later stages of pregnancy you will also be less inclined to suffer shortness of breath if you have maintained good upper back posture. Achieving strong abdominals by training the transversus abdominis muscle will help you to regain a flat stomach more quickly following the birth of your baby.

PELVIC PLACEMENT

The value of correct body alignment cannot be over-emphasized. The tilt of the pelvis affects the alignment of the spine, and both directly affect your entire posture.

Correct pelvic placement creates good posture, which helps you avoid backache and joint strain during pregnancy. Your resulting poise and grace will make you look radiant and feel more confident.

SHOULDER STABILITY

Neck pain and knotty, tense shoulders are common complaints. In pregnancy, extra load is placed on the upper back, shoulders and neck muscles from your increased breast size and growing baby. This causes you to hold your shoulders in a raised and tense position. Pilates targets the appropriate muscles to achieve relaxed shoulders and alleviate neck tension and discomfort.

HEAD AND NECK PLACEMENT

The neck is very susceptible to injury, and the effects of neck damage can be long-lasting, causing pain that fatigues, as well as uncomfortable, restless sleep. Ideally the head needs to be in a well balanced position without any conscious muscular effort. Pilates exercises train you to hold your head and neck correctly to help prevent strain and injury. Correct alignment of the head and neck will add that final flourish to your elegance and poise.

BREATHING TECHNIQUE

To breathe deeply and efficiently, breathe in through your nose and out through your mouth, pursing your lips slightly. When exercising it is essential that you breathe out on the effort of the movement, and breathe in as you relax or prepare for the next movement. This pattern enables you to avoid tension and concentrate fully on each exercise movement. Breathing correctly during exercise encourages your pelvic floor, abdominals and back muscles to connect fully, providing essential stabilization for your pelvis and lumbar spine.

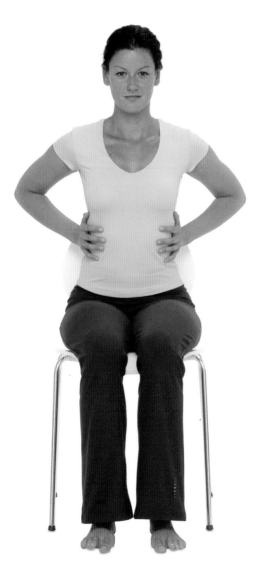

GENTLE HINTS

- Avoid over-breathing. Keep your breathing at a pace you find comfortable to help you avoid breathlessness.

- As your baby grows, particularly in the later stage of pregnancy, breathing deeply may not feel comfortable, so just breathe normally.

- Never hold your breath (many women do this during exercise without realizing) as it may cause dizziness or fainting.

Sit on a stable chair, with your feet flat and hip-width apart. Lengthen upwards through your spine. Place your hands on either side of your ribcage. Breathe in through your nose and feel your ribcage expand sideways into your hands. As you breathe out, feel your ribcage close down.

BREATHING WITH ROLL-DOWN

This breathing exercise incorporates movements that mobilize and release tension in the neck, shoulders and spine. It also encourages the correct use of the abdominal muscles when bending over.

Repetitions: 3

GENTLE HINTS

- Initiate the movement from the top of your head, and focus on feeling your spine roll, vertebra by vertebra, as you move forwards, keeping the movement small.

- As you roll up, initiate the movement from your tailbone.

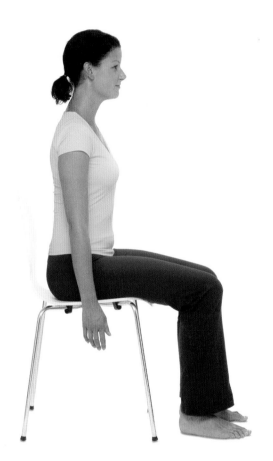

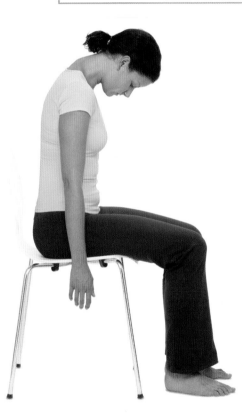

1 Sit on a stable chair, with your feet flat and hip-width apart. Relax your arms down by your sides with your palms facing inwards. Lengthen upwards through your spine. Keep your weight evenly balanced on top of your sit-bones. Gently pull your navel in towards your spine.

2 Breathe in, slowly dropping your chin towards your chest. Breathe out, letting the weight of your head roll you forwards as far as is comfortable, coming to rest in a relaxed position. Breathe in, then pull your navel towards your spine as you breathe out and slowly roll back up, vertebra by vertebra, to an upright position.

Relaxation is vital to ensure that you enjoy your pregnancy. The tranquillity derived from relaxing will transfer its benefits to your growing baby and contribute towards its future health. The relaxation process in this exercise is a series of progressive steps, so you may find it useful to record the sequence, to listen to as you work your way through to perfect relaxation bliss.

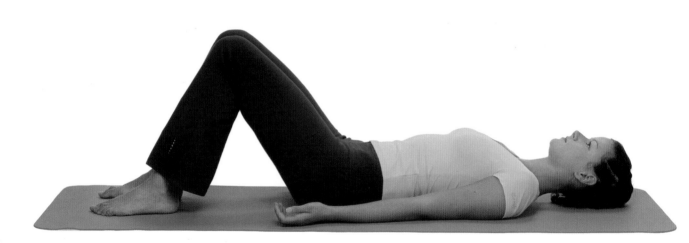

Lie on your back on your exercise mat with your knees bent, feet flat on the floor and hip-width apart. Place a small pillow under your head, if needed. Relax your arms at your sides, with your palms facing up.

- To promote relaxation close your eyes and feel the weight of your feet, pelvis, ribcage, shoulder blades and head lying heavily on your mat. Begin from the tips of your toes and work up your body.
- Imagine your feet as a tripod with three points connecting with the floor – your big toe, little toe and the centre of your heel.
- Keep your knees in a line parallel with your hips. Relax your hip flexors and thighs. If they feel tense, shift your feet further away or closer to your buttocks until they feel comfortable.

- Keep your pelvis in neutral alignment (see 'Neutral spine' on page 36). Imagine your hip bones pointing towards the ceiling. Avoid gripping your buttocks.
- Feel your spine lengthen on the mat.
- Let your shoulder and neck muscles relax, and release any tension in your jaw muscles and face.
- Now feel all the muscles in your body soften. Imagine you are lying on warm sand and are slowly melting into it. Enjoy the sensation of your body in this wonderfully comfortable relaxation position. After three months, practise this in a side-lying position.

The pelvic floor forms an integral part of the central core muscles and plays a vital role in maintaining the body's correct posture. Weak pelvic-floor muscles will lead to poor posture and cause back pain. Lack of proper support for the pelvic organs may lead to a prolapse, a weakness that can cause incontinence or embarrassing leaks when sneezing or laughing, and bladder and bowel problems in later life. Such weakness in the pelvic floor is really not the best preparation for childbirth. Pelvic-floor exercises are probably the most important ones to practise in pregnancy. They also help activate and engage your core abdominal muscles.

TYPES OF MUSCLE FIBRE

The pelvic floor has two types of muscle fibre, known as slow-twitch and fast-twitch. Each type performs a different function and therefore requires a different exercise technique. Approximately two-thirds of the muscles are slow-twitch, performing slow muscle contractions that support the pelvic organs during endurance activities, helping you to stand for prolonged periods while maintaining good posture and enabling you to go for long sessions without 'leaking'. Toning your slow-twitch muscles offers the bonus of heightened sexual pleasure during intercourse. The remaining third of muscle fibres are fast-twitch, which help you retain control when more sudden activities occur, such as jumping, laughing or sneezing. The exercises on the following pages work with the pelvic-floor muscles.

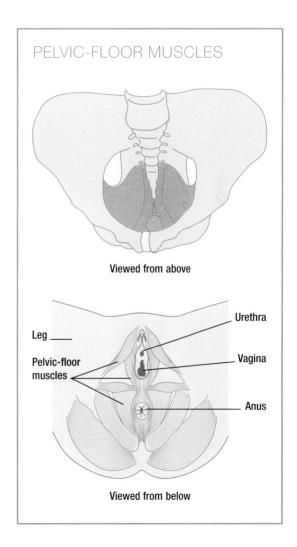

PELVIC-FLOOR MUSCLES

Viewed from above

Leg

Pelvic-floor muscles

Urethra

Vagina

Anus

Viewed from below

PELVIC EXERCISES

The Diamond Lift works the slow-twitch muscles. Extending your 'holding' time provides fantastic toning for the pelvic-floor and sphincter muscles (which assist voluntary control of when to empty the bladder or bowel). The Diamond Pulse works the fast-twitch muscles that prevent embarrassing leaks from sudden sneezes. In late pregnancy, The Big Lift prepares you for the baby's birth.

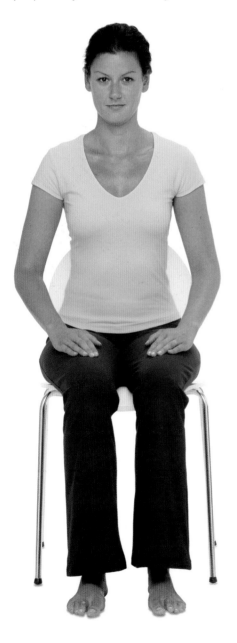

DIAMOND LIFT

Repetitions: 3–5

1 Sit upright on a stable chair, with your feet flat on the floor and hip-width apart. Ensure that your body weight is evenly distributed, with your hips square to the front. Imagine a diamond shape formed by your pubic bone at the front, your sit-bones at each side and your tailbone at the rear. Your pelvic-floor muscles are attached to the four corners of the diamond shape.

2 Breathe in, then breathing out draw the four corners together, pulling inwards and then upwards. Hold for three seconds, then breathe in as you slowly release for six seconds. Lift to bladder level. Feel the transversus muscle contract and engage. Rest for six seconds, then repeat. Gradually increase the hold to ten seconds, with ten seconds rest.

GENTLE HINTS

- Perform frequently throughout the day, or whenever you touch water!

- The drawing in and up action is similar to holding back from breaking wind.

DIAMOND PULSE

Repetitions: 5–10 (three times daily)

Sit on a chair or cross-legged on the floor. Imagine sitting on the four corners of your diamond shape, and quickly 'snatch' those four corners inwards and upwards. Hold for a split second, release rapidly, then relax completely. Repeat.

GENTLE HINTS

- If you anticipate a cough or sneeze coming on, practise this movement immediately before the sneeze.

- Avoid squeezing your inner thighs, gripping your buttocks or tensing your shoulders.

THE BIG LIFT

Repetitions: 3–5

Sit on a chair as for the Diamond Lift, or cross-legged on the floor. Imagine sitting on the four corners of your diamond shape and, as you draw these four corners inwards and upwards, visualize an elevator platform rising to the first floor. Hold the pelvic-floor muscles firmly for two seconds, breathing gently in and out. Now raise the elevator platform to the second floor. Hold for two seconds. Repeat this movement again to the third and fourth floors, holding for two seconds at each level. Slowly release the pelvic floor, lowering one level at a time. Remain in the relaxation phase for eight to ten seconds, then try again.

GENTLE HINTS

- This requires a lot of practice and controlled breathing. At every floor remember to breathe in and out before continuing.

- Stop at the second level if you find this difficult. Progress only when you feel stronger. Later, perform this exercise standing up.

CORE STABILIZATION

The central core refers to the transversus abdominis – the deep-seated band of muscle that wraps itself horizontally around your torso like a corset – the multifidus muscles that support your spine and the pelvic-floor muscles. Strengthening these muscles stabilizes the spine, lumbar spine (lower back) and pelvis. All movements in Pilates are initiated from the central core. To connect and engage these muscles effectively and to promote good stability, practise the following exercises. Avoid lying on your back for longer than three minutes in mid- to late pregnancy.

GENTLE HINTS

- As your abdominal muscles contract, imagine a smile breaking out across your abdomen, spreading from your navel to your spine. Think of it drawing 'back and wide', and of the smile wrapping around your baby!

- Keep your pelvis level and avoid tucking it under.

- Progression: hold the contracted abdominals, breathe in, then out and relax.

CORE CONNECTOR

Repetitions: 2–3

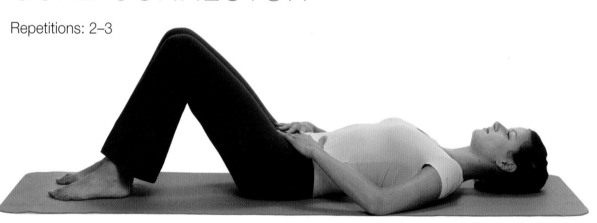

1 Lie on your back with a small pillow under your head, if needed. Place your feet flat on the floor hip-width apart, with your knees bent. Place your palms flat on your hips. Slide your hands 5 cm (2 in) in and 5 cm (2 in) downwards. Spread your fingers, and feel your relaxed abdominals under your fingertips.

2 Breathe into the sides and back of your ribcage. Breathe out and lift your pelvic floor using the Diamond Lift (see page 32). Simultaneously pull your navel in towards your spine. Feel your abdominals move away from your fingertips. Breathe in and release the abdominal muscles. Repeat.

KNEELING CORE CONNECTOR

Repetitions: 5–10

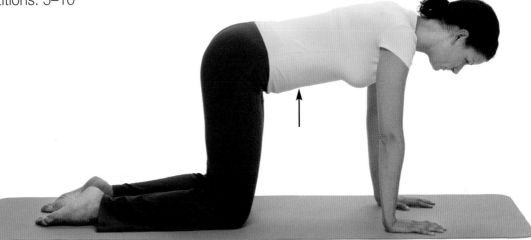

1 Kneel down on all fours, keeping your shoulders over your hands and hips over your knees, with your elbows slightly bent, not locked. Lengthen the top of your head away from your tailbone, maintaining a neutral spine position. Look at the floor, fingertips facing forwards.

2 Breathe into the sides and back of your ribcage. Breathe out, keep your back still and use the Diamond Lift (see page 32) to lift your pelvic floor. Pull your navel in towards your spine. Breathe in to release your abdominals. Repeat.

CORE CONNECTOR WITH BALL

Repetitions: 5–10

Progress this exercise further by placing a small sponge football between your inner thighs. Repeat the Kneeling Core Connector exercise, gently squeezing the ball between your thighs as you lift your pelvic floor up and draw your abdominals towards your spine.

NEUTRAL SPINE

Pilates emphasizes the importance of stabilizing the pelvis and lumbar spine in a neutral position. Understanding how to find this position, and then bringing this awareness to your spinal alignment, is crucial because the tilt of your pelvis affects the alignment of your spine.

GENTLE HINTS

- After three months of pregnancy, avoid lying on your back for longer than three minutes.

- It may help to stand sideways to a mirror and practise this movement.

THE PELVIC ROCKER

Repetitions: as necessary to find the right position

1 Lie on your back with a small pillow beneath your head, if needed. Place your feet flat on the floor, hip-width apart and knees bent. Place your hands on the front of your hips. Tuck your pelvis under, feeling your lower back flatten towards the mat. You will feel your tailbone lift away from the floor and your hip flexors (where the top of your thigh bends) tighten.

2 Gently tilt your pelvis the other way. You will feel a slight arching in your spine. Note: avoid arching your back if you have a back injury.

3 Find your neutral spine by rocking backwards and forwards between these two positions. Neutral lies between these two extremes, where your tailbone drops towards the mat and your pubic bone and hip bones are level. There should be room for a hand to slide between the mat and the back of your waist.

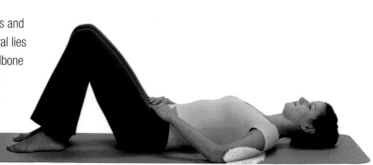

BENT KNEE DROP

Repetitions: up to 3 on each side, alternating

Begin as for The Pelvic Rocker, with your spine in neutral alignment. Place your hands on your hip bones to ensure your hips stay still. Breathe in. As you breathe out, lift your pelvic floor and pull your navel in towards your spine. Let your left knee open outwards. Keep your hips, pelvis and right knee still. Breathe in and return to the start position. Repeat on the other side.

LEG SLIDE

Repetitions: up to 3 on each side, alternating

Begin as for The Pelvic Rocker. Breathe into the sides and back of your ribcage. Breathe out, lift your pelvic floor and pull your navel in towards your spine. At the same time, slide one foot along the mat as far from your buttocks as you can without moving your pelvis. Breathe in and return to the start position. Repeat on the other side.

LYING KNEE LIFT

Repetitions: 3–5 on each side, alternating

Begin as for The Pelvic Rocker. Breathe into the sides and back of your ribcage. Slowly breathe out, lift your pelvic floor and pull your navel in towards your spine. At the same time, float one knee to above the hip at a 90-degree angle. Breathe in, holding the knee lifted while maintaining the abdominal contraction. Breathe out as you slowly lower your foot to the floor. Repeat on the other side.

SHOULDER STABILIZATION

Heavier breasts and the baby's weight may cause neck pain and tense shoulders. These exercises will help to stabilize your shoulder blades and enable you to feel the correct way they should move on your back when initiating arm movements. Arm circles draw attention to ribcage positioning during arm movement.

GENTLE HINT

- After the third month of pregnancy, avoid lying on your back for longer than three minutes and instead try practising the Arm Circles in a standing position.

SCAPULA ISOLATION

Repetitions: 3

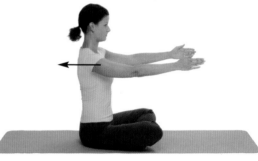

INCORRECT RETRACTED POSITION
Breathe in and gently draw your shoulder blades closer together without forcing them. Breathe out and return to the ideal neutral position. Repeat.

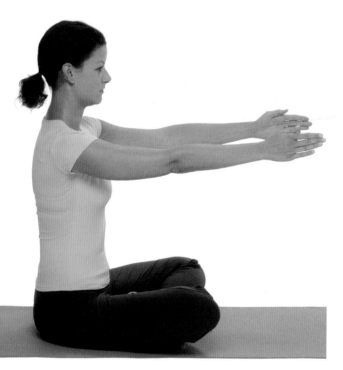

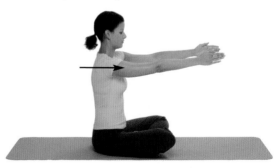

IDEAL NEUTRAL POSITION
Sit tall on your mat with your legs crossed, arms extended in front of you at shoulder level, palms facing and shoulder-width apart. Keep your shoulders relaxed.

INCORRECT PROTRACTED POSITION
Breathe in, stretch and reach forwards with your fingertips. You will feel the gap between your shoulder blades widen. Breathe out and return to the ideal neutral position. Repeat.

SHOULDER SHRUGS AND DROPS

Repetitions: 2 or 3

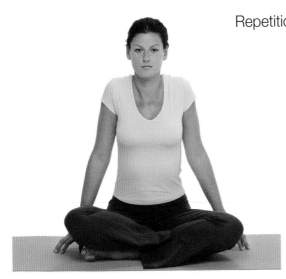
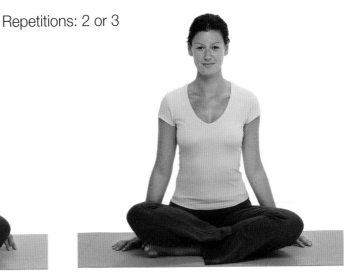

SHRUGS

Sit tall on your mat with legs crossed and arms relaxed by your sides. Breathe in and shrug your shoulders up towards your ears, feeling your shoulder blades slide upwards.

DROPS

Breathe out and slide your shoulder blades down in to your back, pressing your palms lightly into the mat. Breathe in and return to the start position.

ARM CIRCLES

Repetitions: 3 in each direction

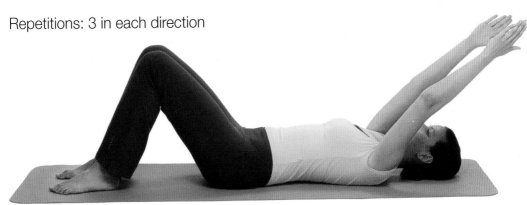

Lie on your back with knees bent and feet flat on the floor, hip-width apart. Raise your arms and stretch your fingertips towards the ceiling. Breathe in to prepare, then breathe out as you pull your navel in towards your spine.

Breathe in and reach your arms overhead, keeping your ribcage in contact with the mat. Breathe out, circling your arms out and round to your hips and returning to the start position.

Pilates teaches you to lengthen the back of the neck, whether lying, sitting or standing, to help you achieve perfect alignment and correct posture. Correct positioning of the head on the neck helps you to avoid discomfort and injury. By balancing the strength of the neck flexors (used to tuck the chin into the chest) and the neck extensors (used for looking up), perfect alignment can be achieved. Your cervical spine will hold its natural curve creating a stronger, healthier posture.

GENTLE HINTS

- Initiate the chin-dropping movement with your eye-line. Look at an imaginary bug on the ceiling and follow its path across the ceiling away from you.

- After the third month of pregnancy, avoid lying on your back for longer than three minutes.

HEAD NODS

Repetitions: 3–5

1 Lie on your back with your knees bent, feet flat on the floor and hip-width apart. Relax your arms by your sides with your palms facing down. Let your body relax, and feel the breadth across your chest.

2 Breathe in and gently drop your chin towards your chest, lengthening the back of your neck without lifting your head off the mat. Breathe out and return to the start position. Repeat.

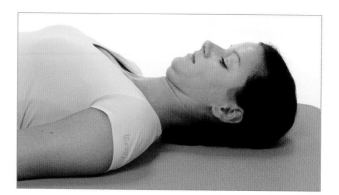

HEAD TILTS

Repetitions: 3 on each side, alternating

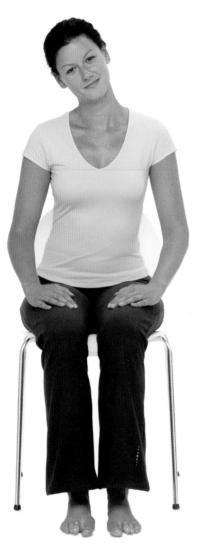

Sit upright on a chair with your stomach pulled in. Position your knees over your feet and rest your hands on your thighs. Keep your eye-line straight ahead throughout, maintaining the breadth across your chest, with your shoulders relaxed. Breathe in and tilt your right ear towards your right shoulder. Return to upright, then tilt your left ear towards your left shoulder. Repeat.

HEAD TURNS

Repetitions: 3 on each side, alternating

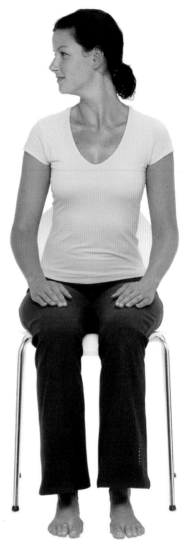

Assume the same start position as for Head Tilts. Turn your head slowly to the right side and hold for a second. Repeat to the left side and hold. Keep your chin level as you turn your head. Repeat.

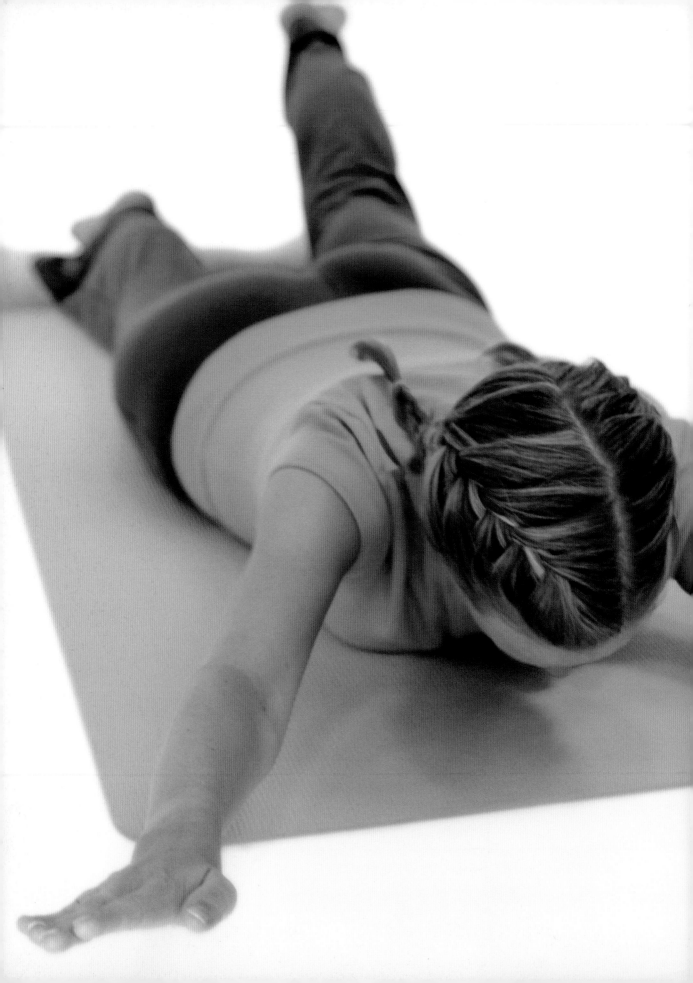

EARLY PREGNANCY
ONE TO THREE MONTHS

CHANGES IN YOUR BODY

Having missed your period and discovered that you are pregnant, you will soon experience emotional and physical changes as your hormones surge. You may feel very emotional, overwhelmed and tire easily. Many women also begin to suffer from sickness or nausea.

Your ligaments and joints are becoming more lax and unstable, which makes you more liable to joint strain or injury and can cause poor posture.

Your waistline gradually expands. If you are keen on exercising and are normally trim, you may find this change alarming, but the weight gain is natural and necessary for your baby to grow.

Rushes of hormones make your breasts enlarge and produce the thin milky secretion known as colostrum in preparation for breastfeeding, and they may feel tender. Your bladder feels the pressure of the growing uterus and you might need to pass water more frequently. Constipation may also begin to trouble you.

Your blood pressure changes, often becoming lower in these early months. These changes sometimes cause you to feel light-headed.

The exercises in this book will lay the foundations for recovering a strong, toned figure after the birth.

GUIDELINES FOR ONE TO THREE MONTHS

- If you are new to Pilates, wait until your pregnancy is established at four months (16 weeks) before starting these programmes – refer to the advice given on page 20.

- If you do need to wait until after your 16th week to commence the exercises, you can still keep fit by taking daily walks to maintain your cardiovascular fitness. Apply the principles of good posture when you walk (see pages 26–27).

- When exercising, perform only as many repetitions as feels comfortable. Don't overdo it!

- Practise your pelvic-floor exercises every day.

- Take care during exercise transitions – move slowly and avoid getting up quickly.

- Pay attention to your technique and your posture. Quality of movement is better than quantity.

- With heavier breasts, there will be a tendency to round your upper back and shoulders, so include lots of Pilates exercises that strengthen your mid-back, such as the Barn Doors exercise (see page 54) and The Kite (see page 60).

- It is important to strengthen and tone your arms and shoulders in preparation for holding, lifting and carrying your baby. The Wall Press (see page 48) combines a super workout for your arms and chest.

- Help avoid constipation by drinking plenty of water and eating at least five portions of fresh fruit and vegetables daily.

- Eating early in the day, and smaller amounts more often, can offset feelings of sickness or nausea. Keep dry crackers to hand as quick hunger fixes.

- If anything feels uncomfortable – STOP!

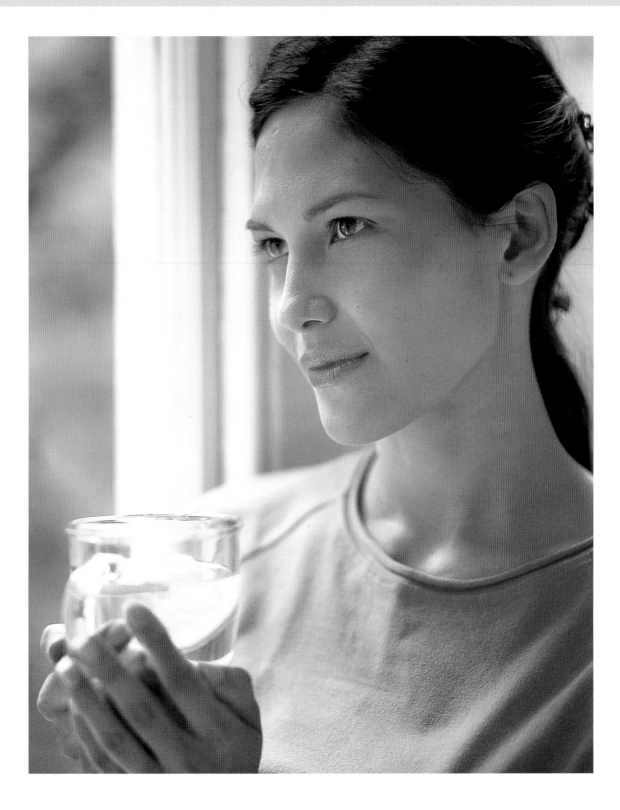

AT-A-GLANCE EARLY PREGNANCY WORKOUT

Perform the full Early Pregnancy Workout at least three times a week. Always prepare by mobilizing the body gently, using the warm-up programme below. This will give you several minutes to increase your self-awareness, focus your mind and awaken your body. Concentration is vital. Clear your mind of the mundane and make this time yours!

AT-A-GLANCE WARM-UP

The warm-up exercises come from the Pilates Basics section (see pages 24–41).
Perform them in the order listed below:

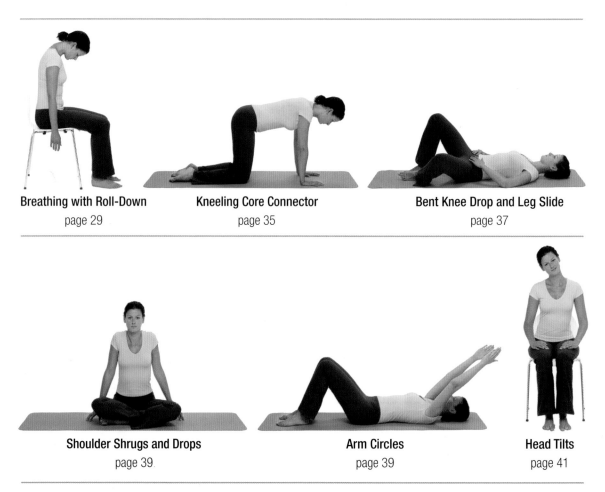

Breathing with Roll-Down
page 29

Kneeling Core Connector
page 35

Bent Knee Drop and Leg Slide
page 37

Shoulder Shrugs and Drops
page 39

Arm Circles
page 39

Head Tilts
page 41

You are now warmed up and ready to begin the Early Pregnancy Workout.
Study the 'At-a-glance exercise sequence chart', then learn the exercises.

AT-A-GLANCE EXERCISE SEQUENCE CHART

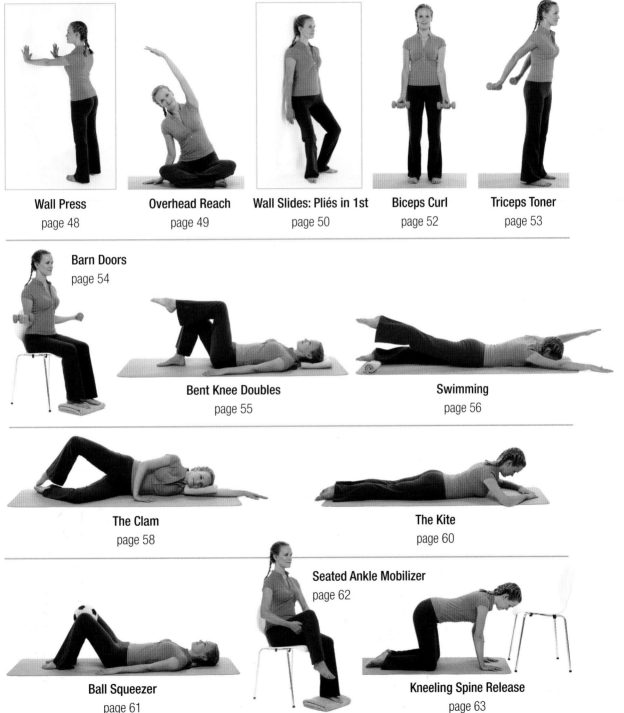

Wall Press
page 48

Overhead Reach
page 49

Wall Slides: Pliés in 1st
page 50

Biceps Curl
page 52

Triceps Toner
page 53

Barn Doors
page 54

Bent Knee Doubles
page 55

Swimming
page 56

The Clam
page 58

The Kite
page 60

Ball Squeezer
page 61

Seated Ankle Mobilizer
page 62

Kneeling Spine Release
page 63

WALL PRESS

The Wall Press is a great exercise for conditioning and toning the muscles at the back of the arm (your triceps) and chest (pectorals). The pectorals lie in front of your shoulders underneath your breasts. Strong pectorals help to support your breasts and provide shape to your décolletage. This wall-based version of the classic press-up is ideal during pregnancy.

Repetitions: 8–10

GENTLE HINTS

- Avoid letting your back sag. Keep your spine lengthened and your stomach held firmly throughout.

- Lead the movement with your chest, not your nose.

- Avoid locking your elbows as you straighten your arms.

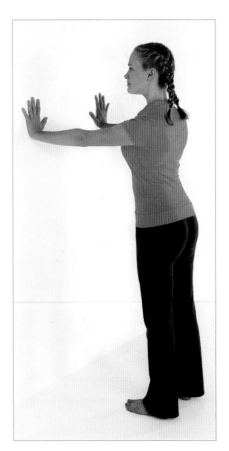

1 Stand tall facing the wall, with your feet hip-width apart and your knees slightly bent. Place your palms flat on the wall in front of you, slightly wider than shoulder-width apart, then step back until your arms are straight.

2 Breathe in and pull your navel in towards your spine. Slowly bend your elbows as you lower your chest towards the wall. Breathe out and press firmly against the wall to return to the start position.

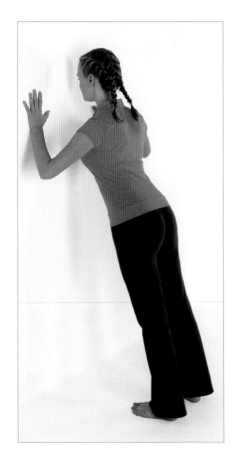

This is a wonderful side-stretch, which is gently effective and feels invigorating to do. The Overhead Reach is performed seated on the floor, so you may feel more comfortable sitting on a large cushion, a yoga block or a rolled-up towel. To ensure a balanced result from this exercise, change the feet crossed in front of you when you alternate sides.

Repetitions: 3–5 on each side

GENTLE HINTS

- Pull your body weight up out of your hips.

- Keep your shoulder relaxed as you raise your arm upwards.

- Keep your head and neck in line with your spine and look straight ahead as you reach over.

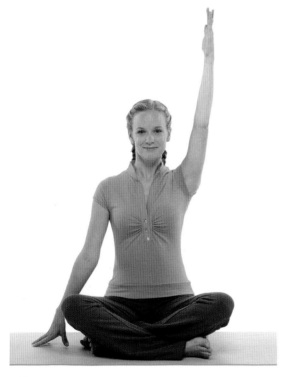

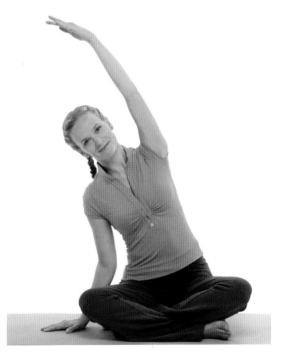

1 Sit comfortably with your legs crossed and pull up tall, lengthening out from the top of your head towards the ceiling. Place your right hand on the floor beside you, and raise your left arm up towards the ceiling, reaching up through your fingertips.

2 Breathe into the sides and back of your ribcage. Breathe out and pull your navel in towards your spine. Lift and lengthen towards the ceiling, then reach across and over with your left arm as far as is comfortable. Keep your hips and shoulders facing the front. Breathe in and pull up through your centre, then return to the start position. Repeat.

WALL SLIDES: PLIES IN 1ST

Pliés originally came from ballet classes, *plier* meaning 'to bend'. These simple knee bends provide excellent tone for all the leg muscles, with the emphasis on the inner thighs and buttocks. Working against the wall helps you pay close attention to core stability and using your abdominal muscles effectively.

Repetitions: 8–10

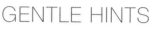

GENTLE HINTS

- Avoid turning your legs out from the knees or ankles.

- If you feel unsure of the turn-out movement, practise the Bent Knee Drops (see page 37).

- Imagine squeezing a coin between your buttocks to help you with the turn-out.

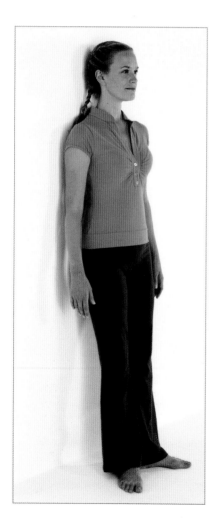

1 Stand with your back against a wall, with your heels about the length of your own foot away from the wall. Place your feet together and gently turn your legs out from the hip joints, keeping your heels as close together as feels comfortable. Look straight ahead.

2 Breathe in. Pull your navel in towards your spine and maintain the contraction throughout the movement. Lengthen through your back, and bend your knees out over your toes as you slide your back down the wall. Do not lift your heels off the floor. Hold for one second, then breathe out as you slide back up the wall to the start position.

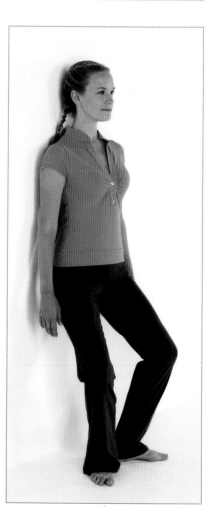

WALL SLIDES: PLIES IN 2ND

When you can perform the Pliés in 1st easily and they no longer present you with a challenge, move on to Pliés in 2nd. These pliés really help you to feel the inner thigh and buttock muscles contracting and working. Pliés will help you achieve toned, shapely legs and a firm bottom.

Repetitions: 8–10

GENTLE HINTS

- Hold your navel in towards your spine throughout the movement.

- If you feel your knees rolling inwards, turn your toes slightly forwards to improve alignment.

- As you straighten back up, squeeze your buttocks together as if trying to grip a coin.

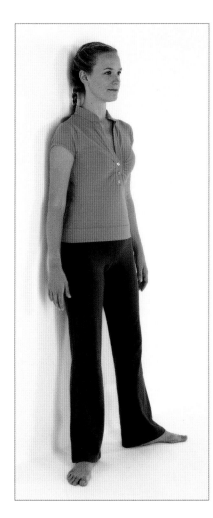

1 Stand with your back against a wall, with your heels about the length of your own foot away from the wall. Place your feet slightly wider than hip-width apart – about 20–25 cm (8–10 in) apart. Slightly turn your legs out from the hip joints. Look straight ahead.

2 Breathing in, pull your navel in towards your spine. Lengthen through your back, and bend your knees out over your toes as you slide your back down the wall. Do not lift your heels off the floor. Hold for a second. Breathe out, squeezing your buttocks and inner thighs as you slide back up the wall to return to the start position.

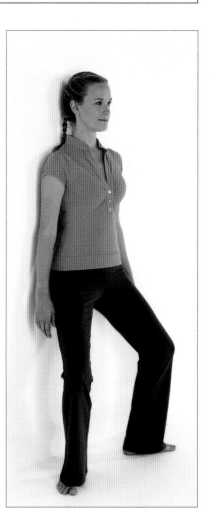

BICEPS CURL

Developing strength in your upper arms helps your back muscles when you perform everyday activities, such as lifting bags and moving furniture when you vacuum. When your new baby arrives, you will be better equipped for all the lifting and carrying that is part of the joy of being a new mum! You will need dumb-bells weighing about 0.45 kg (1lb) or 0.9 kg (2 lb) each for this exercise.

GENTLE HINTS

- Keep your navel pulled in towards your spine throughout to maintain good posture.

- Avoid rounding your shoulders and keep your chest wide.

- This exercise may be performed sitting on a firm, sturdy chair.

Repetitions: 8–10

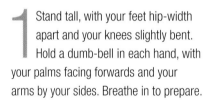

1 Stand tall, with your feet hip-width apart and your knees slightly bent. Hold a dumb-bell in each hand, with your palms facing forwards and your arms by your sides. Breathe in to prepare.

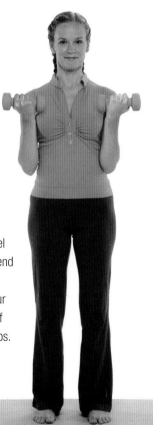

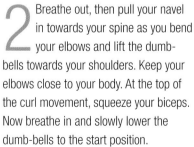

2 Breathe out, then pull your navel in towards your spine as you bend your elbows and lift the dumb-bells towards your shoulders. Keep your elbows close to your body. At the top of the curl movement, squeeze your biceps. Now breathe in and slowly lower the dumb-bells to the start position.

This is an exercise that produces really flattering results. It focuses on strengthening and toning the triceps muscles at the backs of your upper arms. It effectively eliminates flab from this hard-to-reach area, and firms up the backs of your arms so that, when you wave, they don't wobble! You will need dumb-bells weighing about 0.45 kg (1lb) or 0.9 kg (2 lb) each for this exercise.

GENTLE HINTS

- Keep your navel pulled in towards your spine throughout to maintain good posture.

- Slide your shoulder blades gently down your back as you press your arms backwards.

- Avoid arching your upper back.

Repetitions: 8–10

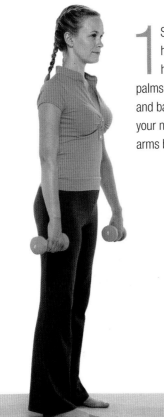

1 Stand tall with good posture, with your feet hip-width apart. Hold a dumb-bell in each hand, with your arms at your sides and your palms facing backwards. Breathe into the sides and back of your ribcage. As you breathe out, pull your navel in towards your spine and push your arms backwards.

2 Hold for a second. Keep your chest area open, maintain good posture and don't let your ribs push forwards. Breathe in and slowly return to the start position. Repeat.

The group of muscles that sit across the shoulder blades plays an important role in overall posture. These muscles must be strengthened to help counteract rounded shoulders and guard against injury. Rounded shoulders cause the chest muscles to tighten, creating muscular imbalance. This exercise is especially helpful for anyone who spends long hours at a desk or driving. The movement helps to encourage you to open the chest area, and promotes awareness of your posture.

GENTLE HINTS

- Use the muscles between the shoulder blades as you move the dumb-bells outwards and keep your shoulder blades down.

- Avoid flexing your wrists.

- This exercise may be performed in a standing position.

Repetitions: 5–10

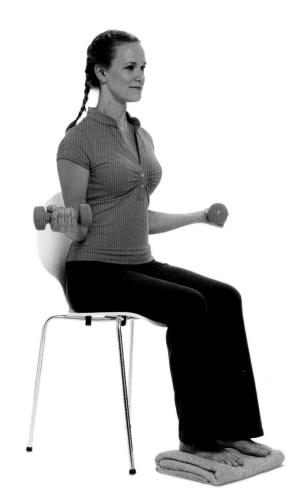

1 Sit comfortably on a sturdy chair, with your feet hip-width apart and your spine in a neutral position. Hold a dumb-bell in each hand and bring your elbows close to your sides at waist level, palms facing up. Breathe in to prepare.

2 Breathe out, pulling your navel in towards your spine to stabilize your back. Keep your elbows close to your sides and move the dumb-bells outwards. Breathe in and return to the start position. Repeat.

BENT KNEE DOUBLES

Maintaining the neutral spine position provides you with a heightened awareness of your transversus abdominis (corset) muscle. This exercise demands good core stability and progresses the benefits you gained from the Lying Knee Lift (see page 37).

Repetitions: 4–6

GENTLE HINTS

- Try not to tense your shoulders.
- Do not allow your lower abdominals to bulge.
- Place a flat cushion below your head for comfort.

1 Lie on your mat, knees bent, feet flat on the floor, hip-width apart. Breathe in. Breathe out, pulling your navel in towards your spine. Float your right knee up above your right hip at a 90-degree angle. Breathe in and place your right hand on your right knee. Breathe out and float the left knee up to a 90-degree angle above the left hip.

2 Breathe in and let go of your right knee. Avoid arching your back. Breathe out and slowly float your right foot to the floor, keeping your navel pulled in towards your spine. Breathe in. Breathe out as you float the left foot to the floor. Repeat, starting each time with the opposite leg.

This is one of the few exercises you do on your stomach and is performed in three stages. It works to strengthen all the back of your body, incorporating your legs, deep buttocks, lower, mid and upper back muscles. It also helps you focus on maintaining a strong centre, using abdominal support when performing movements. The benefits gained all contribute to making you strong and prepared for your pregnancy, the birth and beyond.

Repetitions: 6 of each step, alternating sides

GENTLE HINTS

- Avoid moving your body. Imagine a glass of water balanced on your lower back – keep it still so that it doesn't spill!

- Keep your shoulders relaxed and drawn down your back.

- If your stomach sinks to touch the mat, stop and rest, and start again when you feel refreshed.

- If lying on your stomach is uncomfortable, replace this exercise with Superwoman (see page 78).

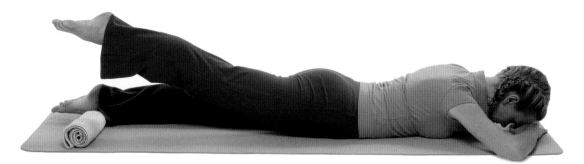

1 Lie face down with a rolled-up towel under your ankles, feet hip-width apart. Rest your forehead on your hands, which should be placed one on top of the other. Find your neutral spine position (see page 36), then lengthen your tailbone away from you. Breathe in and lift your pelvic floor. Pull your navel in towards your spine, lifting your lower abdominals away from the mat. Breathe out and lift your right leg, lengthening your toes away from your tailbone. Breathe in as you lower your leg to the floor.

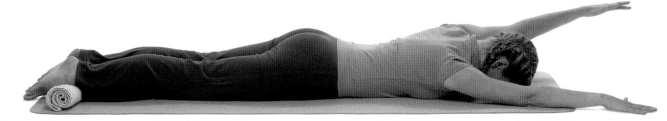

2 Now extend your arms to a V-shape. Breathe in to prepare and, as you breathe out, gently lift your left arm. Breathe in as you slowly lower your arm. Keep your head on the mat and ensure you continue to pull your navel in towards your spine. Alternate arms, keeping your elbows soft and your neck and shoulders relaxed. Repeat.

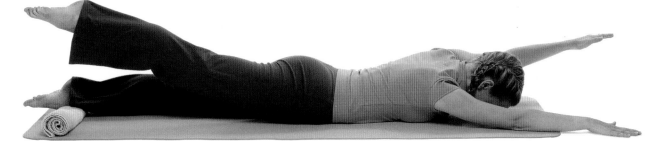

3 Now raise one arm and the opposite leg together, also lifting your head a fraction. Then lower your arm, leg and head to the floor. Lift the other arm and leg, lifting your head slightly. Repeat, ensuring that you keep pulling your navel in towards your spine. Keep the movements low to begin with. As your stomach muscles get stronger, you can lift slightly higher. Your movements must be controlled, lifting your arm and leg to equal height. Only raise your head if you feel strong enough.

THE CLAM

The Clam has many benefits because it works on several different levels. It improves strength in the deep abdominal muscles, providing essential support for your growing baby in the months to follow. It tones and streamlines the muscles of the outer thighs and helps firm the deep-seated buttock muscles. It also enhances stability in your pelvis when your ligaments soften and your body changes during pregnancy. As the name suggests, the leg movements resemble the shell of a clam opening and closing.

Repetitions: 8–10 on each side

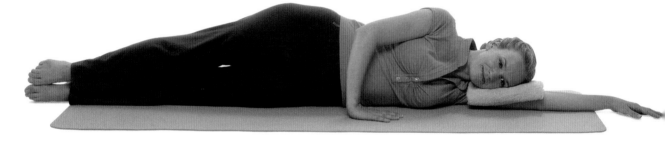

1 Lie on your left side with one hip stacked on top of the other. Straighten your body from head to heels. Place a flat cushion between your head and your left arm, and another beneath your bump if this feels more comfortable. Put your right hand on the floor in front of you at waist level.

GENTLE HINTS

- Avoid letting your hips roll backwards, and keep your waist lifted from the mat.

- Maintain a neutral spine and keep stability in your torso, to avoid movement.

- Concentrate on the outer thigh and buttock muscles.

- Imagine your abdominal muscles hugging the baby.

- Relax your shoulders and keep your movements slow and controlled.

- For a simple alternative, try the Side-Lying Core Connector (see page 97). This will not tone your outer thighs and buttocks, but will give you all the abdominal benefits to help you cope with your baby's increasing weight, and improve your posture.

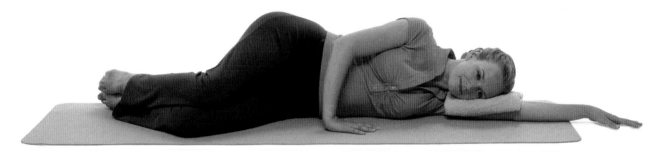

2 Bend your knees forwards until your thighs are at a 45-degree angle to your body. Look straight ahead and breathe in to prepare.

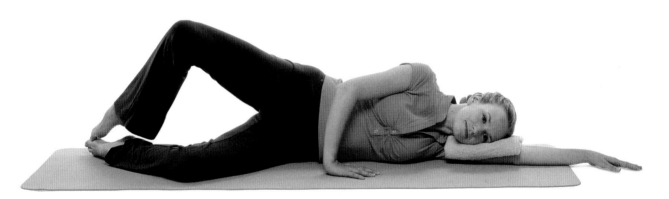

3 Breathe out, pulling your navel in towards your spine. Keep your feet together and open your right knee as far as you can, without your hips rolling backwards. Breathe in as you slowly lower your right knee, returning it to rest on top of your other knee. Repeat.

THE KITE

The Kite looks like a simple exercise, but the effects are really noticeable. It focuses on releasing tension in the mid-upper back and neck muscles. This movement helps to open up the chest area and, as the shoulder blades stabilize and slide down the back, you will feel any tightness in your neck and shoulders just melt away.

Repetitions: 5–10

GENTLE HINTS

- Use your arms for support, but not for pushing up – your back muscles should do the work.

- Avoid looking straight ahead.

- Your upper body lifts only 2.5–5 cm (1–2 in) off the floor. Keep your ribs in contact with the mat.

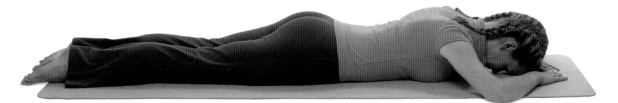

1 Lie on your stomach, with your legs parallel and your feet hip-width apart. Place your palms down, with the tips of your fingers touching and your elbows bent outwards, forming a kite shape with your arms. Relax your neck and shoulders. Breathe in to prepare.

2 Look down as you breathe out, pulling your navel in towards your spine. Lift and lengthen the top of your head away from your tailbone. At the same time as you lift your head and neck into a line with your spine, slide your shoulder blades downwards and draw your chin in slightly. Keep looking at the floor. Breathe in. Breathe out lowering to the start position. Repeat.

BALL SQUEEZER

This is an adaptation of a well-known Pilates exercise that squeezes a ball or pillow. Using a small sponge ball gives a firmer, more positive squeeze. This effective movement combines strengthening the inner thigh muscles with working the pelvic-floor muscles, as well as increasing postural awareness and releasing tension in your lower back. As a bonus, you may also feel your buttock muscles contracting.

Repetitions: 8–10

GENTLE HINTS

- Avoid arching your back as you squeeze the ball.

- If your neck or head feels uncomfortable, place a small cushion under your head.

- If you do not have a sponge ball, use a firm pillow.

1 Lie on your back with your knees bent, your feet flat on the floor and hip-width apart. Hold the ball gently between your knees and rest your arms by your sides, palms facing down. Ensure that your neck and shoulders remain relaxed throughout. Breathe in to prepare, then lift your pelvic-floor muscles.

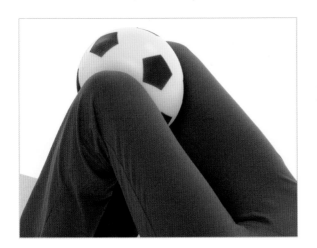

2 Breathe out, pulling your navel in towards your spine, and slowly but firmly squeeze the ball with your knees. Breathe in and hold the squeeze for a second. Then breathe out and slowly relax the squeeze without dropping the ball. Repeat.

SEATED ANKLE MOBILIZER

This is a good movement to practise at the end of a workout or when you are sitting relaxing. It effectively increases ankle mobility and is an efficient way of reducing the swelling in the feet and ankles (oedema) that is so often suffered during pregnancy. It conditions the muscles in the ankles (the flexors and extensors) and improves circulation in the lower limbs by working the calf muscles.

Repetitions: 6 in each direction

GENTLE HINTS

- Maintain good posture throughout, keeping your shoulders and neck free of tension.

- Avoid over-breathing – your breathing should feel relaxed and natural.

- Look straight ahead. If you look down, it will alter your neck and spinal alignment.

1 Sit on a sturdy chair, with your feet flat on the floor and hip-width apart. Maintaining good posture, bend one knee up and hold behind the knee. Breathe normally throughout the exercise.

2 Move the lifted foot clockwise very slowly, completing full circles with each rotation. The movement comes from the ankle joint. Do six clockwise circles, followed by six anti-clockwise circles. Relax, change legs and repeat the movement.

KNEELING SPINE RELEASE

This is an immensely satisfying exercise that gently stretches and releases the spine. It is a kneeling version of the Spine Release (see page 107), which is practised in late pregnancy. The Kneeling Spine Release feels wonderful when used at the end of a workout. You will need a stable chair for support in order to perform this movement.

Repetitions: 1

GENTLE HINTS

- Avoid dipping your back – keep your navel pulled in towards your spine throughout.

- As your spine lengthens, there must be no tension in your shoulder or neck area.

- Enjoy the lovely, long stretch in your spine, through your arms and down into your sides.

1 Kneel down on your mat on all fours in front of your chair's seat, no more than an arm's length away. Keep your knees slightly apart and facing outwards. Your hips should be over your knees and your shoulders over your hands. Breathe in to prepare.

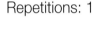

2 Breathe out and walk your hands forward towards the chair seat. Now place your hands palms down and shoulder-width apart on the chair seat. Sit back towards your heels. Hold for up to five seconds, breathing naturally, then release the stretch by placing your hands back on the mat.

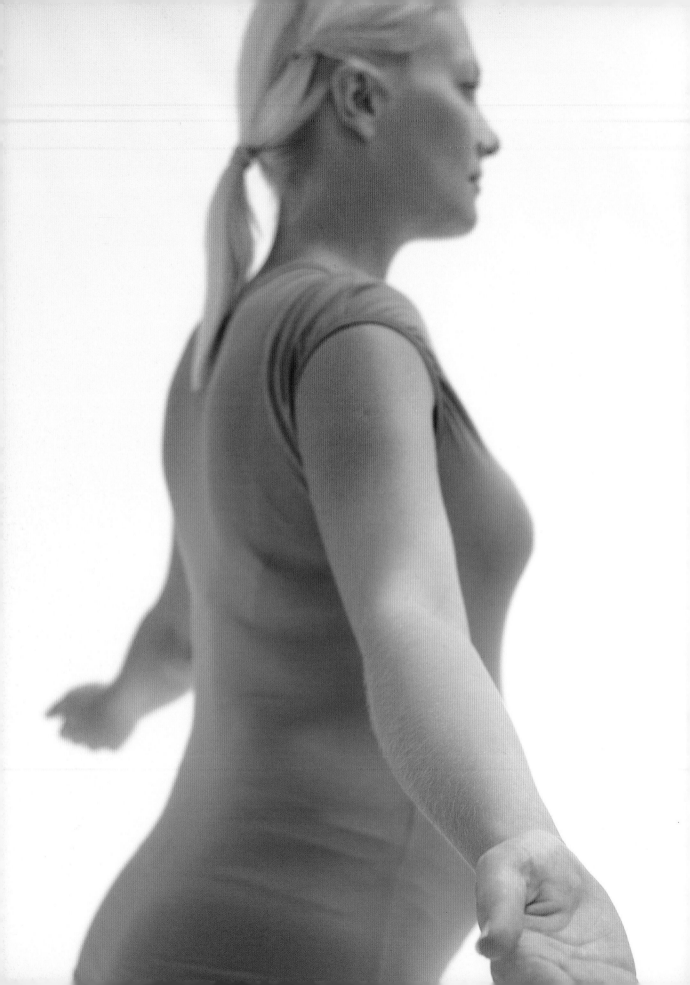

MID-PREGNANCY
FOUR TO SIX MONTHS

CHANGES IN YOUR BODY

You will now find that your posture alters as your baby grows and your tummy becomes rounder. Your shoulders may also start to look more rounded, due to the increasing weight of your breasts. Weight gain will be more noticeable and you may begin to feel self-conscious about your increasing size. However, you will be surprised at how beautiful your growing body looks to everyone around you!

Mid-pregnancy is when you experience most instability in the ligaments and joints around your pelvis. Your rectus abdominis muscles ('the six-pack', see page 12) separate to accommodate your baby's growth.

Fluid retention is more common now. Exercises such as Static Moonwalk (see page 70) and Calf Stretch (see page 76) improve circulation, helping to reduce cramps.

You will be feeling more energetic, and now is the time when you will feel the first exciting movements of your baby inside you, known as 'quickening'.

This amazing experience will give you a real boost! Be careful not to overdo things. A balance of relaxation, exercise and plenty of fresh air will keep you fighting fit and in great form.

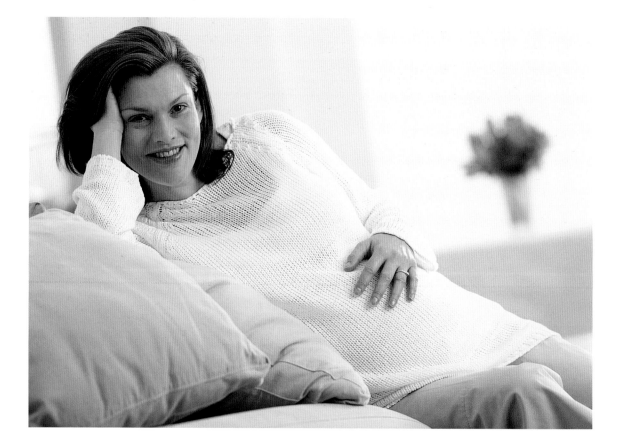

GUIDELINES FOR FOUR TO SIX MONTHS

- Do not spend longer than three minutes lying on your back in any exercise.

- Your larger bump will affect your sense of balance – move smoothly and avoid rushing, particularly when standing up from a lying or seated position.

- Pay attention to your technique and your posture. Quality of movement is more beneficial than quantity.

- Avoid exercising too soon after eating a meal.

- Empty your bladder before starting your Pilates session – you will feel more comfortable and will not need to interrupt your programme.

- Keeping your stomach muscles toned now will help the separated 'six-pack' muscles close within a few weeks after the birth.

- Cease exercising on your front, because it will no longer feel comfortable. The Mid-Pregnancy Workout has alternative exercises to work your back.

- If you feel dizzy or light-headed, lie on your left side and rest until the feeling passes. Have a large cushion nearby so that you can relax comfortably.

- Do your pelvic-floor exercises every day. Each time you touch water, use this as a memory trigger to prompt you.

- Your growing bump will demand more support from your abdominals. Draw your navel towards your spine regularly, even when out walking or queuing at the supermarket checkout. Feel your abdominal muscles wrapping around and lifting your baby.

- When exercising, perform only as many repetitions as feels comfortable. Don't overdo it!

- Keep well hydrated and ensure you drink extra fluids after exercising.

- If you are new to Pilates, you were advised to wait until this stage of your pregnancy before beginning the programme. You must now study Pilates Basics (see pages 24–41) and perform some of the exercises from the Early Pregnancy Workout (see pages 42–63), omitting the two exercises lying on your front, which are Swimming and The Kite, and also omit Bent Knee Doubles and Ball Squeezer. You will then be ready to start the Mid-Pregnancy Workout.

Perform the Mid-Pregnancy Workout at least three times a week. Always prepare by mobilizing the body gently, using the warm-up programme below. This will give you several minutes to increase your self-awareness, focus your mind and awaken your body. Concentration is vital. Clear your mind of trivial everyday thoughts and devote this time to yourself.

AT-A-GLANCE WARM-UP

The warm-up exercises come from the Pilates Basics section (see pages 24–41).
Perform them in the order listed below:

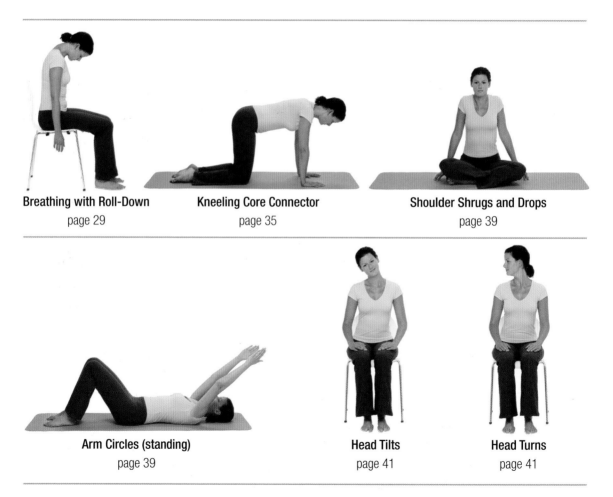

Breathing with Roll-Down
page 29

Kneeling Core Connector
page 35

Shoulder Shrugs and Drops
page 39

Arm Circles (standing)
page 39

Head Tilts
page 41

Head Turns
page 41

You are now warmed up and ready to begin the Mid-Pregnancy Workout.
Study the 'At-a-glance exercise sequence chart', then learn the exercises.

AT-A-GLANCE EXERCISE SEQUENCE CHART

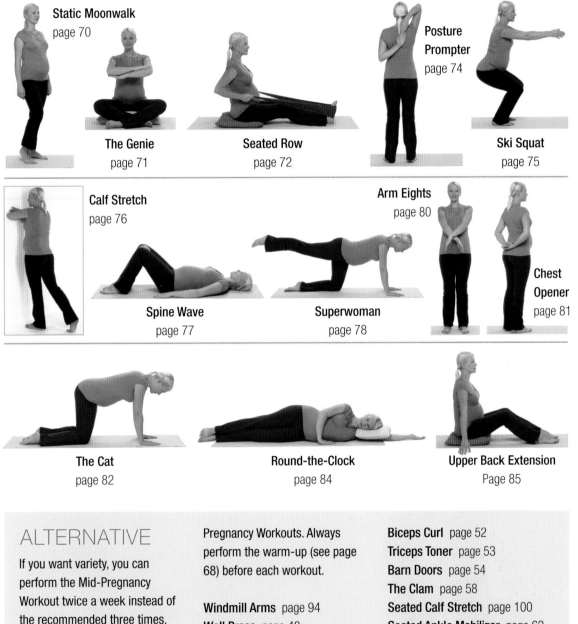

Static Moonwalk
page 70

The Genie
page 71

Seated Row
page 72

Posture Prompter
page 74

Ski Squat
page 75

Calf Stretch
page 76

Arm Eights
page 80

Spine Wave
page 77

Superwoman
page 78

Chest Opener
page 81

The Cat
page 82

Round-the-Clock
page 84

Upper Back Extension
Page 85

ALTERNATIVE

If you want variety, you can perform the Mid-Pregnancy Workout twice a week instead of the recommended three times. Replace the third workout with the exercises below, which have been selected from the Early and Late Pregnancy Workouts. Always perform the warm-up (see page 68) before each workout.

Windmill Arms page 94
Wall Press page 48
Overhead Reach page 49
Wall Slides: Pliés in 1st page 50

Biceps Curl page 52
Triceps Toner page 53
Barn Doors page 54
The Clam page 58
Seated Calf Stretch page 100
Seated Ankle Mobilizer page 62
Kneeling Spine Release page 63

A simple exercise with many benefits, the Static Moonwalk is very beneficial for the circulation during pregnancy. This movement strengthens your feet, calves and thigh muscles, with the bonus of enhanced balance and coordination. Static Moonwalk is an invigorating exercise for mid-pregnancy and is the ideal booster to set you up for your workout.

Repetitions: 20

GENTLE HINTS

- If you find it difficult to balance, hold the back of a sturdy chair for support.

- Keep your hips level, your pelvis still and avoid any jerky movements.

- Lengthen through your spine, concentrating on good body alignment and slow, controlled and flowing movements.

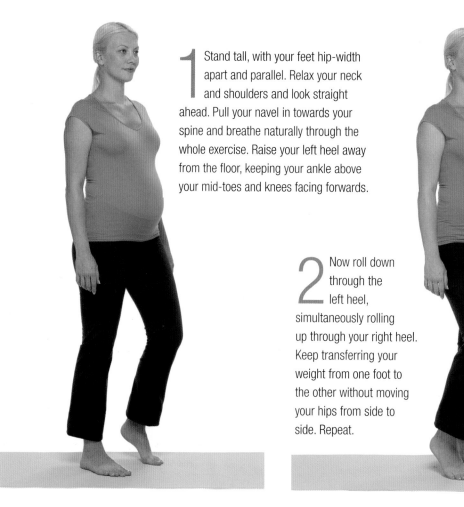

1 Stand tall, with your feet hip-width apart and parallel. Relax your neck and shoulders and look straight ahead. Pull your navel in towards your spine and breathe naturally through the whole exercise. Raise your left heel away from the floor, keeping your ankle above your mid-toes and knees facing forwards.

2 Now roll down through the left heel, simultaneously rolling up through your right heel. Keep transferring your weight from one foot to the other without moving your hips from side to side. Repeat.

THE GENIE

The Genie works on improving mobility in the upper back area. You will be able to feel the muscles in your back gently stretching and working as you perform this turning movement. Resting your fingers on your elbows encourages you to relax your shoulders and helps you to focus on stabilizing the shoulder blades.

Repetitions: 5 on each side

GENTLE HINTS

- Keep your hips facing the front as you turn.

- Feel the breadth across your chest and soften your shoulders.

- Imagine a broom handle placed down your spine, to help you sit tall and lengthen your back.

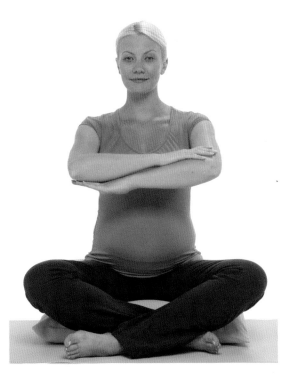

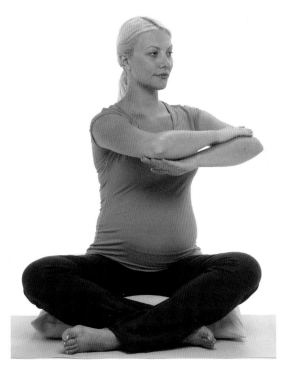

1 Sit cross-legged on a cushion so that your weight is forward into your pelvis. Rest your fingertips on your elbows, and one arm on top of the other. Pull up tall from the top of your head towards the ceiling, and gently draw your shoulder blades downwards. Breathe in to prepare.

2 As you breathe out, pull your navel in towards your spine and turn your upper body to the left side. Keep your chin in line with the centre of your arms. Breathe in as you return to the start position. Repeat to your right side. Continue alternating between your left and right sides.

SEATED ROW

This super exercise really enables you to feel the muscles of the mid-back working, at the same time helping to keep your arms in great shape. It will strengthen the muscles that you will be using for tasks such as getting your baby out of the car seat and carrying him or her in front of you. Keeping these muscles strong will also guard against injury from all the awkward lifting and carrying, and will prevent you from slouching and adopting harmful postural habits. Perform the standard version or the variation – do not do both. You will need an exercise band.

Repetitions: 10

GENTLE HINTS

- Caution: avoid-arching your back. Remember to use your stomach muscles and keep your spine in a neutral position.

- If you do not have an exercise band, perform the exercise by visualizing the resistance.

- Imagine drawing your elbows back through thick mud.

- Keep the movement low, relaxing your neck and shoulders.

- Draw your elbows back in a straight line, parallel with each other, as if on railway tracks.

1 Sit tall on a cushion so that your weight is forward into your pelvis, keeping your knees parallel and slightly bent. Place the centre of the band under the middle of both feet. Hold each end of the band firmly. Breathe in to prepare, then pull your navel in towards your spine and lengthen upwards through your back.

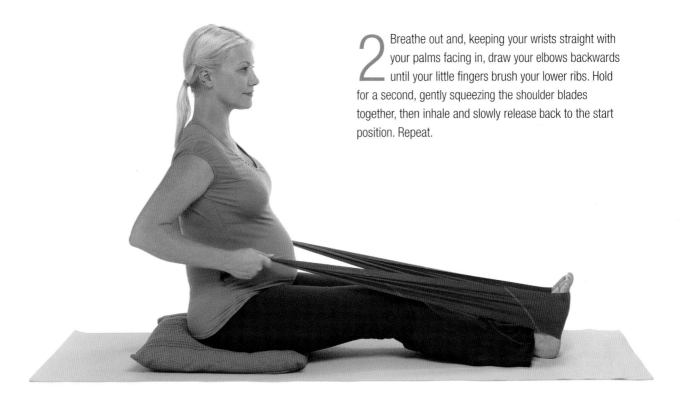

2 Breathe out and, keeping your wrists straight with your palms facing in, draw your elbows backwards until your little fingers brush your lower ribs. Hold for a second, gently squeezing the shoulder blades together, then inhale and slowly release back to the start position. Repeat.

VARIATION

For a variation on the Seated Row, adopt the same start position, but this time keep your palms facing up towards the ceiling. Do not flex your wrists. Your hands should remain in this position throughout the exercise. Perform the same rowing movement as described in step 2. Repeat.

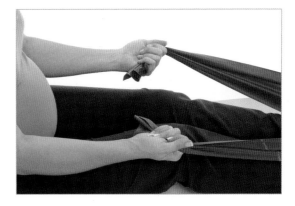

This exercise feels so good that you will want to do it every day. It focuses on your shoulders, chest and upper back, preventing tension and stiffness in these areas and releasing tight muscles. Practise it regularly to promote good posture and avoid a hunched upper back and rounded shoulders.

Repetitions: 1 on each side

GENTLE HINTS

- Maintain good posture throughout the exercise and avoid arching your lower back.

- Keep the shoulder of your raised arm relaxed.

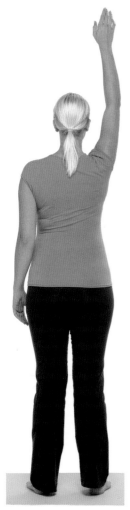

1 Stand tall, with your feet parallel and hip-width apart. Look straight ahead with your chin level. Breathe in, then breathe out as you pull your navel in towards your spine. Breathe in and lengthen your back as you float your right arm above your head.

2 Breathe in, then breathe out as you bend your right arm backwards and reach down your spine with your hand. Breathe in and reach your left hand behind you from below and try and join the fingertips of both hands together. Hold for six to eight seconds, breathing normally. Release the hold. Repeat on the other side.

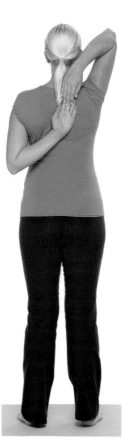

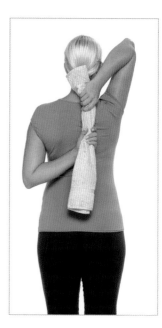

VARIATION

As a variation, use a rolled-up towel or scarf if your hands won't touch. Progressively walk your lower hand up the towel.

SKI SQUAT

Squatting is a practical and functional movement to practise during mid- to late pregnancy. The Ski Squat opens the pelvis to help prepare for the birth. It provides good tone for the thigh muscles and buttocks, and helps strengthen the back. The combined arm reaches help you to concentrate on the shoulder-blade connection. This is a simple and effective exercise that you should practise regularly.

GENTLE HINTS

- Maintain good alignment of your head and neck.

- As you squat, imagine the top of your head lengthening away from your tailbone.

- Bend your knees directly over the centre of each foot.

Repetitions: 6–8

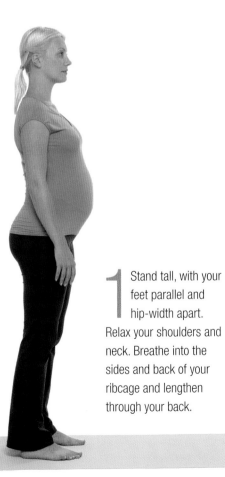

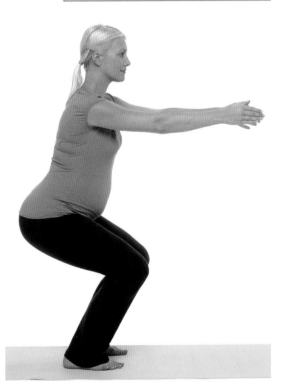

1 Stand tall, with your feet parallel and hip-width apart. Relax your shoulders and neck. Breathe into the sides and back of your ribcage and lengthen through your back.

2 Breathe out, pull your navel in towards your spine. Maintain this contraction throughout. Bend your knees, pivoting forwards from your hips, and simultaneously reach both arms forward to chest level until you reach a comfortable squatting position. Breathe in, squeeze your buttocks and rise to the stand tall position, lowering your arms as you straighten. Repeat.

This stretch is good for knotty calves, releasing tension in the muscles. Whether you have been walking a lot, working out or simply finding that your calves are becoming more prone to cramp, this is a satisfying stretch to perform any time. Well-stretched calves also have the advantage of being more resistant to injury.

Repetitions: 1 on each side

GENTLE HINTS

- Gently press your hips towards the wall to achieve a good stretch.

- Keep your knees, hips and toes facing forwards.

- Breathe naturally throughout.

- Use this stretch as often as you want to in daily life.

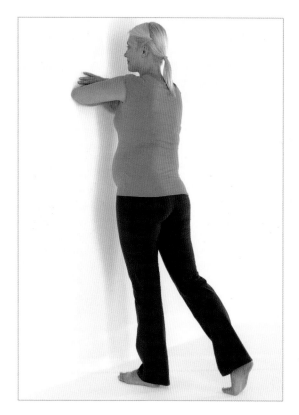

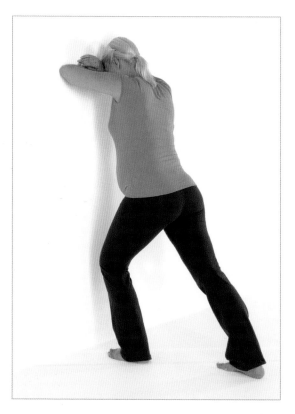

1 Facing a wall, bend your elbows and place your hands and forearms, shoulder-width apart, against the wall. Bend your left knee and position your right leg behind you on the ball of your foot. Pull your navel in towards your spine throughout the movement.

2 Now press your right heel into the floor, allowing your weight to fall forwards onto your arms. Your toes should point forwards. Hold this position for eight to ten seconds, feeling the stretch in your right calf. Relax, then repeat on the other side.

SPINE WAVE

This superb exercise mobilizes your back and releases tension. The Spine Wave not only encourages spinal mobility, but also works your pelvic floor and tones your abdominal muscles, as well as strengthening the muscles of your hamstrings, buttocks and inner thighs. You will need a softball or rolled-up towel between your knees and a flat cushion under your head if needed.

Repetitions: 3–5

GENTLE HINTS

- Visualize each section of your spine as you roll up. As you roll down, imagine that your spine is a car tyre rolling the imprint of its tread into your mat.

- Lift only the lower part of your spine off the mat.

- Keep all of your movements small and controlled.

- Initiate the movement by contracting your abdominals.

1 Lie on your back with your knees bent, your feet flat on the floor and hip-width apart. Place the softball between your knees. Position your arms by your sides with palms facing down. Keep your shoulders soft throughout. Breathe into the sides and back of your ribcage and lengthen through your spine.

2 Breathe out, gently pressing the softball with your knees as you lift your pelvic floor and pull your navel in towards your spine. Squeeze your buttocks and slowly curl your tailbone off the floor, vertebra by vertebra, lifting to a height that is comfortable. Breathe in, hold this position for a second, then breathe out as you slowly lower back to the start position.

SUPERWOMAN

Superwoman is a first-class exercise for strengthening the lower back, and is a variation on the Swimming exercise (see page 56) used in early pregnancy. This effective all-round exercise targets your lower, mid- and upper back and uses your deep buttocks and lower abdominals to help you stabilize and balance. Start with the arms-only version (steps 1 and 2) before moving on to the legs-only version (step 3). When you can perform both of these versions comfortably, progress to the arm and leg combination (step 4).

Repetitions: 6 of each version

(see page 56)

GENTLE HINTS

- When you lift your arm and/or leg, do not lean your body weight over onto the supporting side.

- Avoid lifting or dropping your hips.

- Imagine that your back is a table top with a glass of water on it, which you don't want to spill!

- Avoid transferring your body weight over to one side.

- Try to visualize your lower abdominal muscles wrapping around your baby.

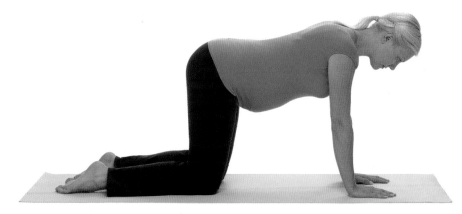

1 For the arms-only version, kneel on all fours, with your hands directly under your shoulders, your knees hip-width apart and under your hips. With your back in a neutral spine position, lengthen the top of your head away from your tailbone and drop your shoulders away from your ears. Look down at the floor.

2 Breathe into the sides and back of your ribcage. Breathe out, pulling your navel in towards your spine, and extend and lift your right arm, palm facing down, until it is parallel to the floor. Breathe in and return to the start position. Repeat with the left arm.

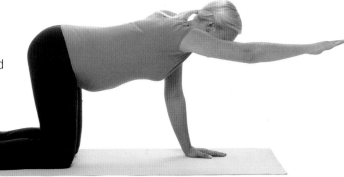

3 Legs-only: Breathe in. Breathe out, pulling your navel in towards your spine, and extend and lift your right leg until it is parallel to the floor. If you feel unsteady, lift your leg just a little way off the floor. Breathe in and return to the start position. Repeat with the left leg.

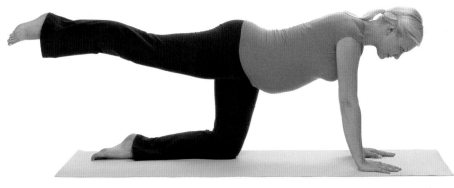

4 Arm and leg combination: Breathe in. Breathe out, pulling your navel in towards your spine, and simultaneously extend and lift your right arm and left leg until they are parallel to the floor. Keep your neck long. Breathe in and slowly return to the start position. Repeat with the left arm and right leg.

This brilliant exercise really helps tone up the wobbly area at the backs of the arms. It sculpts the whole upper arm and shapes the shoulders to provide lean definition. It is very easy to do and requires no equipment. It is a movement adapted from dance classes, and will help you to tighten and firm up unsightly, flappy arms in no time.

GENTLE HINTS

- Keep your shoulders down and away from your ears.

- Ensure you change the way that your palms face correctly, as this is vital to achieve the correct toning effect.

Repetitions: 10

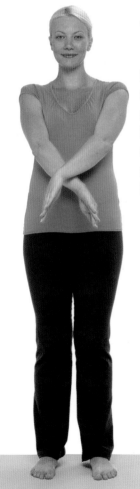

1 Stand tall, with your arms relaxed by your sides and your feet hip-width apart. Pull your navel in towards your spine and lengthen the top of your head towards the ceiling. Breathe in, bringing your arms across in front of you, with your palms slightly apart and facing each other.

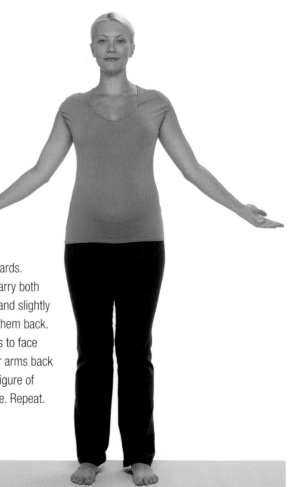

2 Turn your palms upwards. Breathe out as you carry both your arms outwards and slightly behind you, without forcing them back. Breathing in, turn your palms to face backwards as you carry your arms back in front of you. Imagine the figure of eight that your arms describe. Repeat.

This movement reduces the build-up of tension in the shoulders and upper back muscles and will help to improve your posture. It produces a lovely stretch and an open feeling across the chest area. Practised regularly, it will help to combat rounded shoulders and prevent tight pectoral muscles. Do this when you have been bent over a computer or desk for too long.

GENTLE HINT

- If you find it uncomfortable clasping your hands behind you, hold a rolled-up towel between your palms, with your hands 5–7.5 cm (2–3 in) apart.

Repetitions: 1

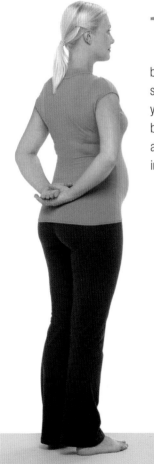

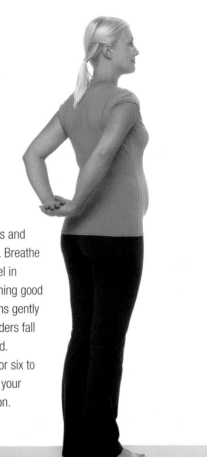

1 Stand tall, with your feet hip-width apart and your weight evenly distributed between both feet. Relax your shoulders, neck and jaw. Bring your hands behind your lower back and gently clasp one hand around the other, without interlinking your fingers.

2 Breathe into the sides and back of your ribcage. Breathe out, pulling your navel in towards your spine, maintaining good posture and raising your arms gently up and back. Let your shoulders fall open and look straight ahead. Breathe naturally and hold for six to eight seconds. Slowly lower your arms and release the position.

THE CAT

Visualize the sinuous, sensual and deeply satisfying stretch of a cat when practising this exercise. It's an excellent movement to enhance spinal mobility and can often help alleviate back pains and aches. The increasing weight of your baby often forces your lower back into an arch. Kneeling on all fours offsets this, easing the pressure on your lower back.

Repetitions: 3–5

GENTLE HINTS

- Visualize the stretch rippling up through your spine, keeping the movement smooth and controlled.

- Relax your shoulders so that they do not hunch up to your ears.

- Avoid locking your elbows – keep them soft.

- Never hollow out your lower back. Always start and finish the exercise with a neutral spine.

- Keep your weight evenly placed between both hands.

1 Kneel on all fours, with your hands directly under your shoulders and your knees under your hips and hip-width apart. Look down at the mat. Lengthen the top of your head away from your tailbone and keep a neutral spine position. Gently slide your shoulder blades down into your back.

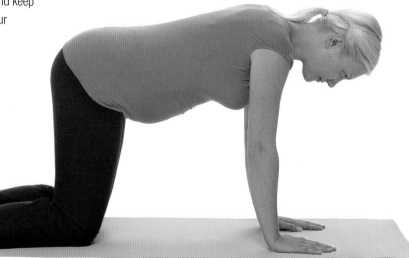

2 Breathe into the sides and back of your ribcage. Breathe out and pull your navel in towards your spine. Initiate the movement by curling your tailbone. Then slowly work the stretch up through your spine from your tailbone, vertebra by vertebra, to your neck and head. As the stretch reaches your neck, point the top of your head down towards the floor. Breathe in. Leading the movement from your tailbone, slowly uncurl your spine, sliding the shoulder blades down into your back as you return to the start position with a neutral spine.

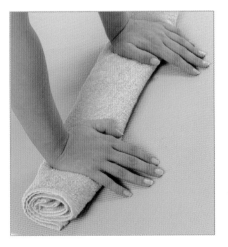

VARIATION

If you find this exercise hard on your wrists or suffer from carpal tunnel syndrome, try resting the heels of your hands on a rolled-up towel. This helps to reduce the angle of your wrists. As your baby grows bigger you may prefer simply to breathe on all fours, in which case practise the Kneeling Core Connector (see page 35).

This is an amazingly comfortable position to exercise in as your baby's weight increases. Round-the-Clock uses a movement adapted from the dancer's workout of circling the leg, but here uses small controlled circles, which not only firm the buttocks, but also tone the inner and outer thighs – a perfect movement to target those hard-to-reach areas during pregnancy.

GENTLE HINTS

- Keep your hips facing to the front.
- Place a cushion between your head and arm.
- The shoulder of your supporting arm must remain relaxed.

Repetitions: 5 clockwise, 5 anti-clockwise on both sides

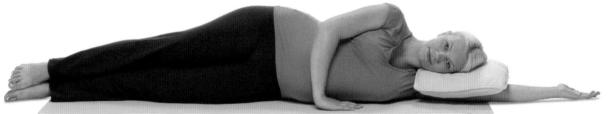

1 Lie on your left side, with one hip stacked on top of the other. Straighten by forming an imaginary line through your ear, the middle of your shoulder, your hip and your ankle. Stretch your left arm above your head, palm facing up, and rest your right arm in front of you.

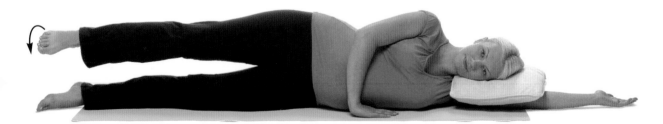

2 Breathe in. Breathe out, pulling your navel in towards your spine. Slowly lift your right leg, raising your foot to hip height. Breathing naturally, draw five compact circles with your foot in each direction. Repeat on your other side.

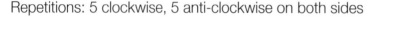

UPPER BACK EXTENSION

As your baby grows bigger, you can no longer lie comfortably on your stomach, but everyday jobs such as vacuuming or gardening compel you to bend forwards. Balance this constant forward bending with this exercise that opens the chest and extends the upper back, without working the lower back.

Repetitions: 4–8

GENTLE HINTS

- Avoid tilting your chin right up.

- Your ribcage must not pop forwards. Ensure that your navel is pulled in towards your spine throughout this exercise.

1 Sit tall on a cushion with your knees bent, your feet flat on the floor and placed a comfortable width apart. Position your fingertips on the floor, out to your sides. Breathe in and lengthen upwards through your spine.

2 Breathe out, pulling your navel in towards your spine, and lift your upper chest towards the ceiling, simultaneously sliding your shoulder blades down into your back. Allow your eye-line to follow a natural path, tracking from straight ahead to the top of the wall. Hold the position as you breathe in. Breathing out, slowly lower back to the start position. Repeat.

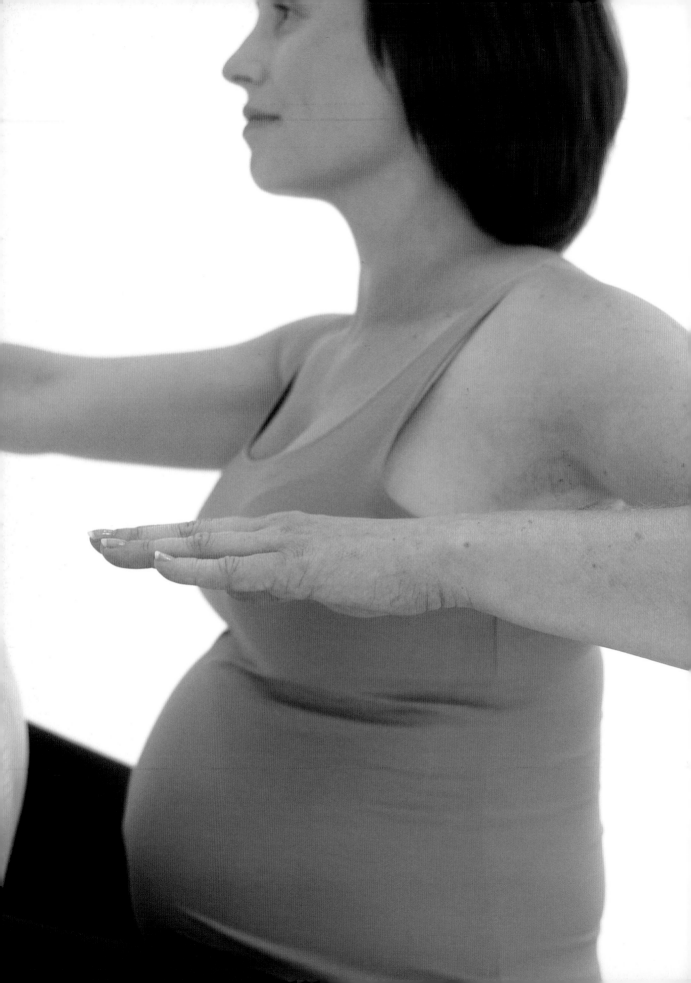

LATE PREGNANCY
SEVEN TO NINE MONTHS

CHANGES IN YOUR BODY

By now your growing baby is fitting more snugly inside your uterus. This may be cosy for baby, but you feel more awkward and uncomfortable as you experience consistent weight gain until around 36 weeks.

Changes in your posture and how you walk are more exaggerated and this is the most common time to suffer lower back pain and discomfort. Hormone levels are keeping your joints loose, making good body alignment and correct posture even more important. At around 28 weeks onwards your breasts may start to leak colostrum and you may start to experience rehearsal contractions.

The expansion in your uterus can cause pressure against your diaphragm, leading to shortness of breath.

The Pilates breathing patterns you have learnt should certainly help alleviate this.

Many women find that their concentration levels deteriorate and short-term memory hits an all time low. With your hormones running amok and your mind diverted by your baby it is hardly surprising!

You are now in a precious preparation time. Use it wisely. Set aside rare moments to enjoy the luxury of being at one with yourself. Do something indulgent, and look forward to the arrival of your new baby.

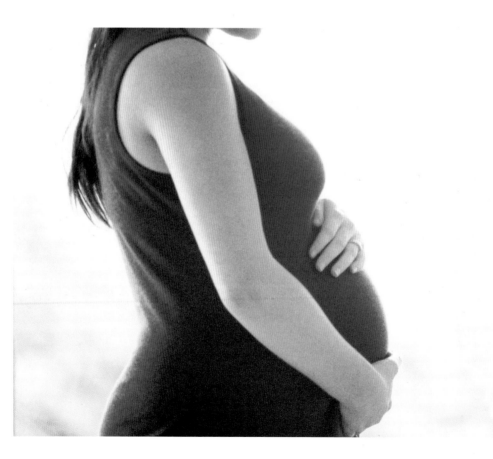

GUIDELINES FOR 7 TO 9 MONTHS

- Ask your doctor or midwife at every ante-natal check to confirm that you are still able to continue your Pilates exercises.

- During each exercise transition avoid hurrying. Come up from lying down smoothly and slowly, see pages 18–19. Do not over exert yourself or become tired or breathless.

- Avoid exercising too soon after eating a meal. Especially important in order to avoid heartburn and indigestion.

- Empty your bladder before starting your Pilates session – you will be more comfortable and will not need to interrupt your programme.

- If you experience rehearsal contractions when exercising, stop if they make you uncomfortable. Whilst they do you no harm, they may put you off.

- Do your pelvic floor exercises every day. Try using each time you touch water as a memory trigger to prompt you. Particularly helpful in preparation for the birth is the Diamond Release on page 96.

- Be aware of your posture. Stand tall, walk with poise and pull your navel towards your spine. The Pilates postural exercises selected for you in late pregnancy are aimed at working the muscles between the shoulder blades to prevent rounded shoulders and to strengthen the mid-back muscles.

- Sit on a cushion or rigid foam block when seated on the floor.

- Exercises which promote better circulation, such as Seated Ankle Mobilizers on page 62, Static Moonwalk on page 70, and Tip & Dip on page 95, should be practised regularly.

- Stretches for your calf muscles feel great and help avoid cramps. Use the Calf Stretch on page 76, and the seated version on page 100.

- Pay attention to your technique and posture. Quality of movement is more beneficial than aiming at quantity.

- To help prepare you for giving birth, practise Wall Squats, see page 102. In this position the pelvis opens and the head of your baby presses down. In the lead up to the birth this is a useful movement.

- Avoid consecutive standing exercises or holding stretches longer than the recommended time in each position.

- If you suffer from swollen fingers or hands then using Tension Tamers on page 103 will help to alleviate this problem.

- If something hurts, STOP. This is your body's way of telling you something is not right.

- Do not spend longer than three minutes lying on your back in any exercise.

AT-A-GLANCE LATE PREGNANCY WORKOUT

Perform the Late Pregnancy Workout three times a week, or at least once a week when combined with two other workout sessions (see pages 92–93). Always prepare by mobilizing the body gently, using the warm-up programme below. This will give you several minutes to increase your self-awareness, focus your mind and awaken your body. Concentration is vital. Clear your mind of the mundane and make this time yours.

AT-A-GLANCE WARM-UP

The warm-up exercises come from the Pilates Basics section (see pages 24–41). Perform them in the order listed below:

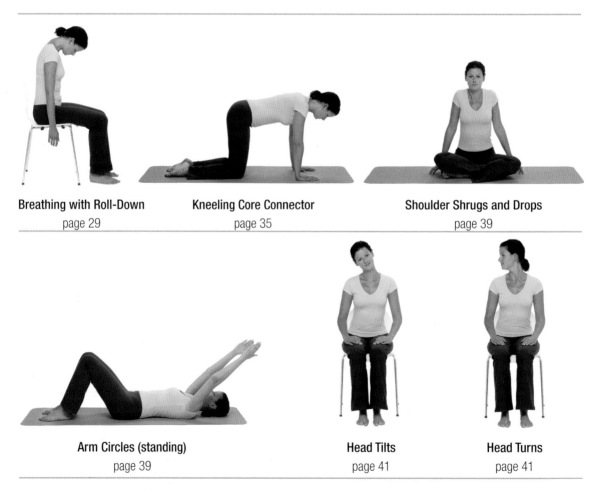

Breathing with Roll-Down
page 29

Kneeling Core Connector
page 35

Shoulder Shrugs and Drops
page 39

Arm Circles (standing)
page 39

Head Tilts
page 41

Head Turns
page 41

You are now warmed up and ready to begin the Late Pregnancy Workout.
Study the 'At-a-glance exercise sequence chart', then learn the exercises.

AT-A-GLANCE EXERCISE SEQUENCE CHART

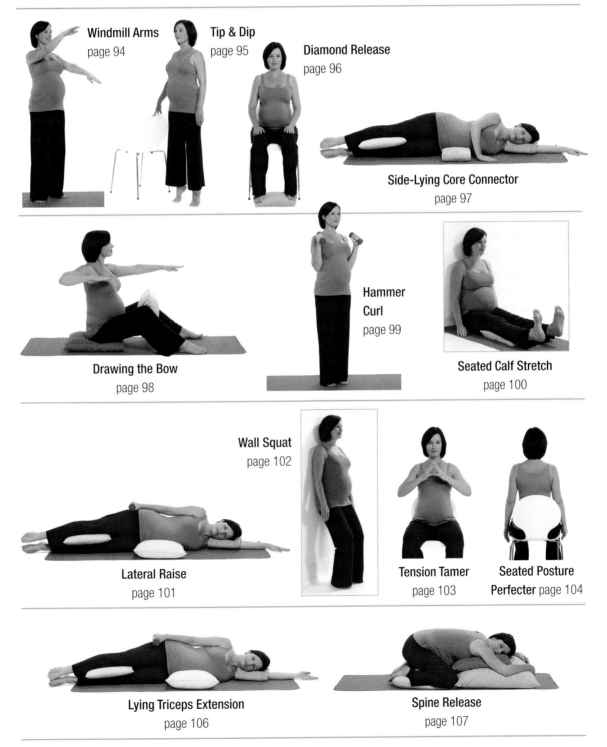

Windmill Arms page 94

Tip & Dip page 95

Diamond Release page 96

Side-Lying Core Connector page 97

Drawing the Bow page 98

Hammer Curl page 99

Seated Calf Stretch page 100

Lateral Raise page 101

Wall Squat page 102

Tension Tamer page 103

Seated Posture Perfecter page 104

Lying Triceps Extension page 106

Spine Release page 107

ALTERNATIVE WORKOUT

You are now going to be spoilt for choice with your Pilates exercises. You have the opportunity to choose your own favourite mix of exercise programmes. At this point you might be feeling big and cumbersome and may tire more easily, so keep yourself motivated and stimulated by putting together a balanced plan from the following suggestions. Check that you still have your doctor's consent to keep exercising, and bear in mind that every session is making you fit and strong in preparation for your baby's arrival. Remember, too, that you will regain your figure much more quickly after the birth if you exercise now.

Opposite are two workout choices based on your exercises to date. You can mix-and-match workouts as long as you ensure that at least one of your weekly sessions is the Late Pregnancy Workout (see page 91). However, do not mix exercises from different workouts because each programme is balanced. But you could, for example, perform Workout One on day one; rest for a day and then perform Workout Two; rest for another day and then do the Late Pregnancy Workout, to complete your three exercise sessions for the week. Or you may decide to do all three weekly sessions using the Late Pregnancy Workout – the choice is yours. Always prepare by mobilizing the body gently, using the six warm-up movements from Pilates Basics (see pages 24–41) that you have been practising before starting your workouts. They are shown again on page 90. Perform them in the order listed.

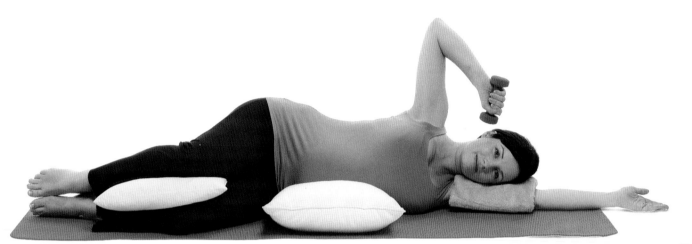

WORKOUT ONE

WORKOUT TWO

WINDMILL ARMS

This exercise will help to enhance your posture and will enable you to focus on releasing tension in your neck and shoulder muscles. As the name suggests, the fluent and relaxed movement of your arms emulates the paddles of a windmill. Windmill Arms provides a lovely overture to your Late Pregnancy Workout.

Repetitions: 8–10

GENTLE HINTS

- Pull your navel in towards your spine throughout the exercise.

- Avoid arching your back.

- Relax your neck and keep your shoulder blades down in your back.

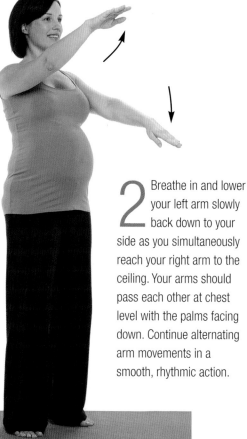

1 Stand tall, placing your feet hip-width apart, with your toes, knees and hips facing forwards. Lengthen upwards through your spine. Relax your arms by your sides, with your palms facing backwards. Breathe in and then breathe out, pulling your navel in towards your spine. Reach your left arm to the ceiling with your palm facing forwards, keeping your right arm still.

2 Breathe in and lower your left arm slowly back down to your side as you simultaneously reach your right arm to the ceiling. Your arms should pass each other at chest level with the palms facing down. Continue alternating arm movements in a smooth, rhythmic action.

TIP & DIP

Tip & Dip incorporates mimic squats and heel raises and will raise awareness of good body alignment. This multi-functional exercise enhances the strength in the fronts of the legs, helping to stabilize the knees while providing a good stretch for your calves. It will also assist in improving the circulation.

Repetitions: 8–10

GENTLE HINTS

- Avoid sticking your bottom out.
- Concentrate on keeping good balance and smooth movements.

1 Stand beside a sturdy chair, placing your feet hip-width apart and maintaining good posture. Rest one hand on the back of the chair for support, if necessary. Breathe into the sides and back of your ribcage. Breathing out, lengthen your spine and bend your knees while keeping your heels flat on the ground.

2 Breathe in and straighten your knees. Breathing out, pull the top of your head towards the ceiling and rise up onto your tiptoes. Aim your tailbone towards the floor. Breathe in and lower to the start position. Repeat.

This is an exercise for your pelvic floor and a variation on The Big Lift (see page 33), which taught you how to lift and lower the pelvic-floor muscles like an elevator. The Diamond Release now takes the elevator platform on past the ground floor and down to the cellar! Practising this now is a vital part of the preparation for your baby's birth. Be sure to go to the toilet before you start, as this is going to teach you how to let go of your pelvic floor completely.

Repetitions: 5–8

GENTLE HINTS

- This is not a difficult movement, but, as with the other pelvic-floor exercises, it needs regular practice in the run-up to labour and birth.

- Persevere: the Diamond Release will help you learn to release the pelvic floor at crucial stages.

Sit tall on a stable chair. Rest your palms on your thighs and place your feet flat on a folded towel, block or phone directory, hip-width apart. Practise The Big Lift as before, taking the elevator platform to the top floor. When you release to the ground level, relax and then release to the cellar. It will take a little practice to relax sufficiently to release completely and fully let go. Repeat.

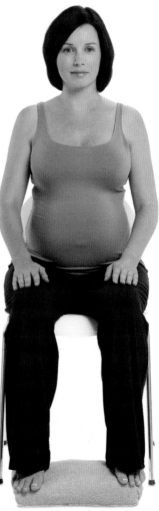

SIDE-LYING CORE CONNECTOR

A variation of the Core Connector (see page 34), this side-lying version is ideal for practising in the latter stages of pregnancy to promote and improve core stability. It will strengthen the muscles that stabilize the spine, lower back and pelvis. With your baby and you reaching the heaviest phase of pregnancy, it is even more important now that you provide good support for your bump and lower back.

(see page 34)

GENTLE HINTS

- Avoid lifting the shoulder of your supporting arm.

- Your waist should not sink down.

- Use two or three cushions or folded towels to support you during this exercise.

Repetitions: 2–3

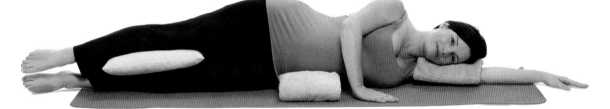

1 Lie on your left side, with one hip stacked on top of the other. Straighten your body from head to heel. Place a folded towel between your head and your left arm, another beneath your bump and one between your knees. Put your right hand on the floor in front of you at waist level.

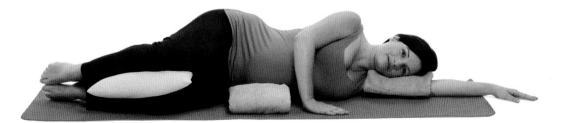

2 Bend your knees forwards until your thighs are at a 45-degree angle to your body. Breathe in to prepare. Breathe out as you lift your pelvic floor and draw your navel in towards your spine. Breathe naturally and hold on to your abdominal contraction for three to five breaths. Relax.

DRAWING THE BOW

A gentle exercise, this helps you practise lengthening through the body as you rotate your spine. Working the muscles of the waist, it also helps to open the upper body while using a slow, controlled turning movement. Perform this exercise sitting on a cushion for comfort and hold a cushion between your knees.

Repetitions: 5 on each side

1 Sit tall on your sit-bones with your knees bent and your feet a comfortable width apart. Place a cushion between your knees to help maintain good pelvic alignment. Hold your arms in front of you at shoulder level, with the palms facing down.

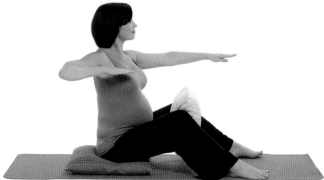

2 Breathe in, keeping your shoulder blades down and your neck relaxed. Now breathe out and pull your navel in towards your spine. Breathe in, bending your right elbow to bring your right hand in towards your chest, in the action of drawing a bowstring back.

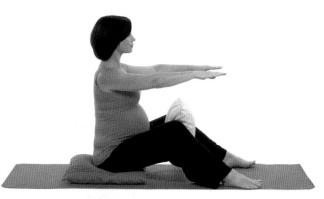

3 Now continue unfolding your right arm to extend it diagonally behind you. Your eyes should follow your moving hand. Squeeze your knees together. Breathe out and bring your arm in a wide arc back to the start position. Repeat four times and then change sides.

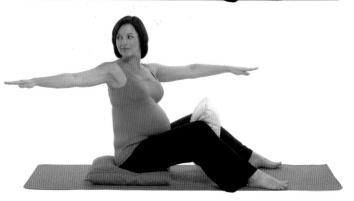

HAMMER CURL

The Hammer Curl is a variation on the Biceps Curl (see page 52), with the accent on toning and defining the outer part of your upper arms. It will make your arms look leaner and longer, and sculpted arms look sexy! The Hammer Curl will produce enviable results. You will need dumb-bells weighing about 0.45 kg (1 lb) or 0.9 kg (2 lb) each for this exercise.

Repetitions: 6–10

> ## GENTLE HINTS
>
> - Avoid locking your elbows as you straighten your arms.
>
> - Do not swing your arms as you lift and lower, otherwise momentum carries you through instead of your biceps working.

1 Stand tall, holding a dumb-bell in each hand. Position your elbows close to your sides, with your palms facing in. Place your feet hip-width apart, with your knees slightly bent. Breathe in, lengthening upwards through your spine.

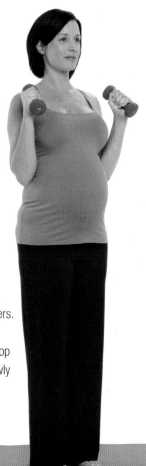

2 Breathe out, pulling your navel in towards your spine, and lift the dumb-bells towards your shoulders. Keep your elbows close to your sides as you lift and squeeze your biceps at the top of the movement. Breathe in as you slowly lower to the start position. Repeat.

SEATED CALF STRETCH

This is a functional exercise very well suited to the late stages of pregnancy. When the risk of oedema (fluid retention) increases, the Seated Calf Stretch will not only help prevent cramping calves, but will also improve the range of motion in your ankles and ease tired, swollen feet. A side-benefit is a boost to the circulation in your legs.

Repetitions: 8–10

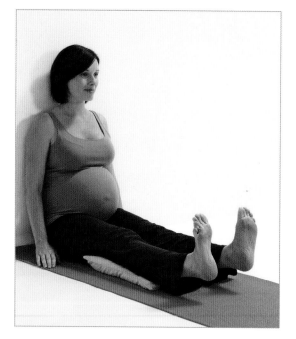

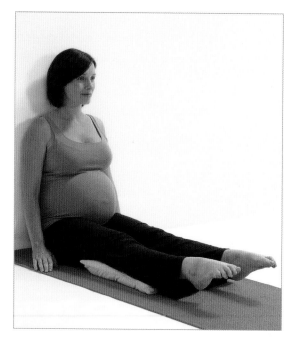

1 Sit on the floor, with your back positioned against a wall. Place a large cushion under both knees for support. Push your heels outwards and flex your toes up to the ceiling. Hold for two seconds.

2 Now point your toes down towards the floor and hold for two seconds. Repeat by alternately flexing the toes up and then down.

LATERAL RAISE

This excellent arm exercise tones the muscles of the mid-shoulder. With a lot of long-term lifting ahead, strength in this area is essential. The mid-shoulder muscle performs the task of stabilization when you are lifting heavier objects and, with a new-born baby rapidly gaining weight, you will want to be fully prepared. Select a 0.45 kg (1 lb) dumb-bell for this exercise.

Repetitions: 6–10 on each side

GENTLE HINTS

- If you find that you roll backwards, lie against a wall.

- To avoid rotating your shoulder, keep the inside of your arm facing downwards.

- Keep your navel pulled in towards your spine throughout.

1 Lie on your left side, with one hip stacked on top of the other. Straighten your body from head to heels. Place a flat cushion between your head and your left arm, another beneath your bump and one between your knees. Hold the dumb-bell in your right hand, resting it on the outside of your right thigh.

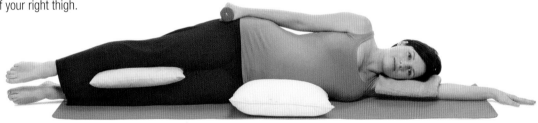

2 Bend your knees forwards until your thighs are at a 45-degree angle to your body. Slightly bend your left elbow, keeping it in line with your body. Breathe in and then, breathing out, slowly lift the dumb-bell, raising your arm to form a 45-degree angle with your body. Breathe in and slowly lower down to the start position. Repeat.

WALL SQUAT

The Wall Squat is one of the most effective exercises you can perform. Great for all-round strength in the thighs, buttocks and lower back, this movement also stretches the calf muscles and enhances your posture. It helps you to concentrate on lengthening the bottom of the spine and on good pelvic alignment. Squatting is also beneficial for the pelvis in preparation for the birth.

GENTLE HINTS

- Keep lengthening your tailbone away from you.
- Keep your navel pulled in towards your spine throughout.

Repetitions: 6–10

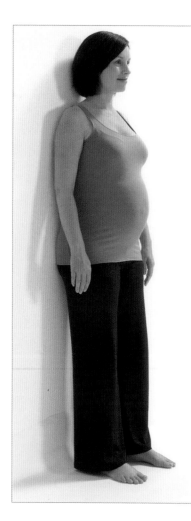

1 Stand with your back against the wall, with about 15 cm (6 in) between your heels and the wall. Place your feet hip-width apart, with your knees and toes facing forwards. Lean into the wall, without putting your head against it, and relax your shoulders and neck.

2 Breathe into the sides and back of your ribcage. Breathe out, pulling your navel in towards your spine. Now, breathing normally, bend your knees and slide a little way down the wall. Slide smoothly back up again to the start position. Note: slide only a little way down or you will not get up again!

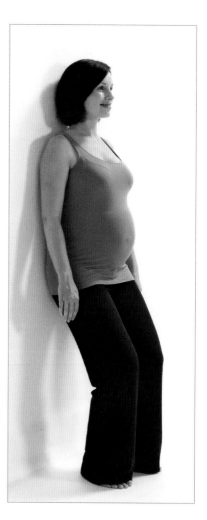

TENSION TAMER

This exercise helps counteract the effect of fluid accumulation in pregnancy. Oedema is usually a swelling of the feet and ankles caused by fluid retention in the body during pregnancy. The condition can, however, also affect the hands and wrists. If you suffer from swollen fingers, this is a simple and effective exercise that you can perform anywhere.

Repetitions: 1 x 8-second hold (step 1), 8 (step 2)

GENTLE HINTS

- Relax your neck and shoulders.

- Place a yoga block or folded towel beneath your feet if they don't quite touch the ground.

1 Sit upright on a chair and place your fingertips together in front of you at chest level. The heels of your hands should not be touching each other. Press the tips of your fingers firmly against each other. Breathe naturally and hold the press for eight seconds. Release and shake out your hands below waist level, releasing tension.

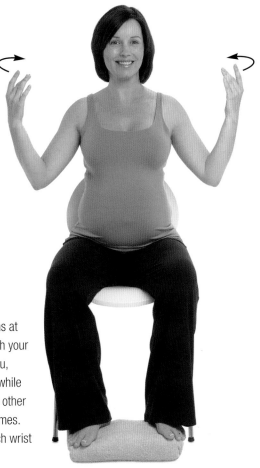

2 Now bend your arms at the elbows and, with your hands in front of you, circle one wrist clockwise while simultaneously circling the other wrist anti-clockwise four times. Repeat four times with each wrist in the opposite direction.

SEATED POSTURE PERFECTER

The Posture Perfecter is the perfect exercise to target the muscles of the upper back. This subtle movement, effectively reduces backache, improving the way you hold yourself. The benefits to your posture are clearly visible. If your feet don't quite touch the floor, place a folded towel, firm cushion or yoga block beneath them.

Repetitions: 6

GENTLE HINTS

- Look straight ahead, keeping your neck in line with your spine.

- As you squeeze your shoulder blades together, feel the muscles between your shoulder blades contracting.

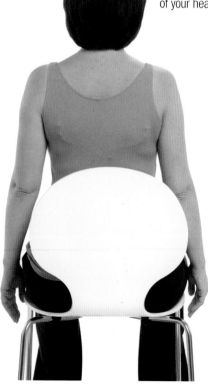

1 Sit tall on a chair with your feet flat on the floor, hip-width apart. Keep your arms relaxed at your sides. Imagine a cord attached to the top of your head, pulling you up towards the ceiling.

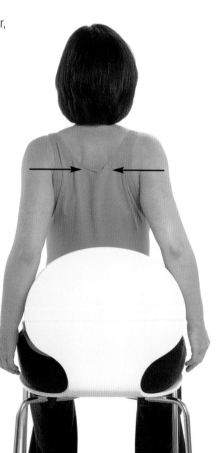

2 Breathe in and then breathe out, pulling your navel in towards your spine. Hold this contraction throughout. Breathing naturally, gently squeeze your shoulder blades together. Hold the squeeze for three to four seconds, then release to the start position. Repeat.

The standing version of the Posture Perfecter (step 1) is especially useful when standing at the supermarket checkout or queuing at the bank! There is also a simple variation (step 2), which works the same area, but also enables you to work the large muscles at the sides of your back that stabilize the upper body.

Repetitions: 6 of each step

GENTLE HINTS

- Concentrate on feeling the large muscles at the sides of your back being worked.

- Keep your forearms parallel and at the same level as you move them back and forth – do not allow them to drop.

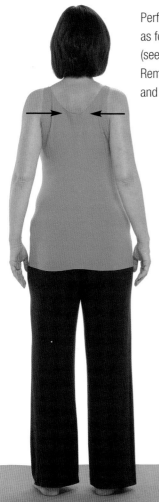

Perform exactly the same exercise as for the Seated Posture Perfecter (see opposite), but in a standing position. Remember to keep your shoulders soft and your neck relaxed.

VARIATION

For the variation, stand tall with good posture, with your feet hip-width apart and your knees and toes facing forwards. Raise your arms out to the sides at shoulder level, then bend your elbows to a 90-degree angle, with your forearms parallel and palms facing down. Pull your navel in towards your spine and, breathing naturally, slide your elbows backwards without moving your shoulders, and then return your arms to the start position. Repeat.

LYING TRICEPS EXTENSION

Targeting the triceps muscles at the backs of the arms, this exercise is a comfortable way of working the upper arm muscles. It will tone wobbly arms, keeping them functionally strong for carrying and lifting your baby. Use several cushions for support and one 0.45 kg (1 lb) dumb-bell.

Repetitions: 6–10 on each side

GENTLE HINTS

- Avoid locking your elbow as you straighten your arm.

- When holding the dumb-bell, do not flex your wrist.

- Pull your navel in towards your spine throughout.

1 Lie on your left side, with one hip stacked on top of the other. Straighten your body from head to heels. Place a folded towel between your head and your left arm, another beneath your bump and one between your knees. Hold the dumb-bell in your right hand, resting it on the outside of your right thigh.

2 Bend your knees forwards until your thighs are at a 45-degree angle to your body. Breathe in and bend your right arm, positioning your hand beside your ear, with your elbow pointing towards the ceiling. Breathe out, pulling your navel in towards your spine, and lift the dumb-bell towards the ceiling. Breathe in and lower to the start position. Repeat.

The Spine Release lengthens the spine and provides a complete stretch for the whole back. It helps relieve pressure and ease tension in the upper and lower back, and assists in opening the pelvis. Do the Spine Release whenever you have backache, or after a workout or tiring day. You will need several large cushions.

Repetitions: 1

GENTLE HINTS

- Soften all your muscles and relax your joints.

- Visualize yourself lying on warm sand and melting into it. Enjoy this relaxing sensation.

- You may find that playing relaxing music will help you to unwind.

1 Place some large cushions on the floor in front of you. Kneel on another cushion, keeping your knees slightly apart, with your feet close to your buttocks. Relax your neck and shoulders.

2 Position your hands on the floor in front of you and walk your hands out towards the cushions. Place your head and arms on top of the cushions and relax, turning your head to the side and lengthening your spine. Breathe naturally and hold for a minute. Return carefully to the start position.

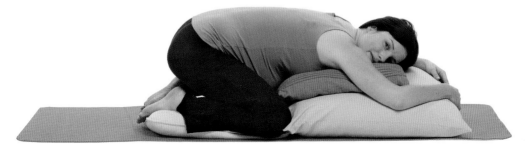

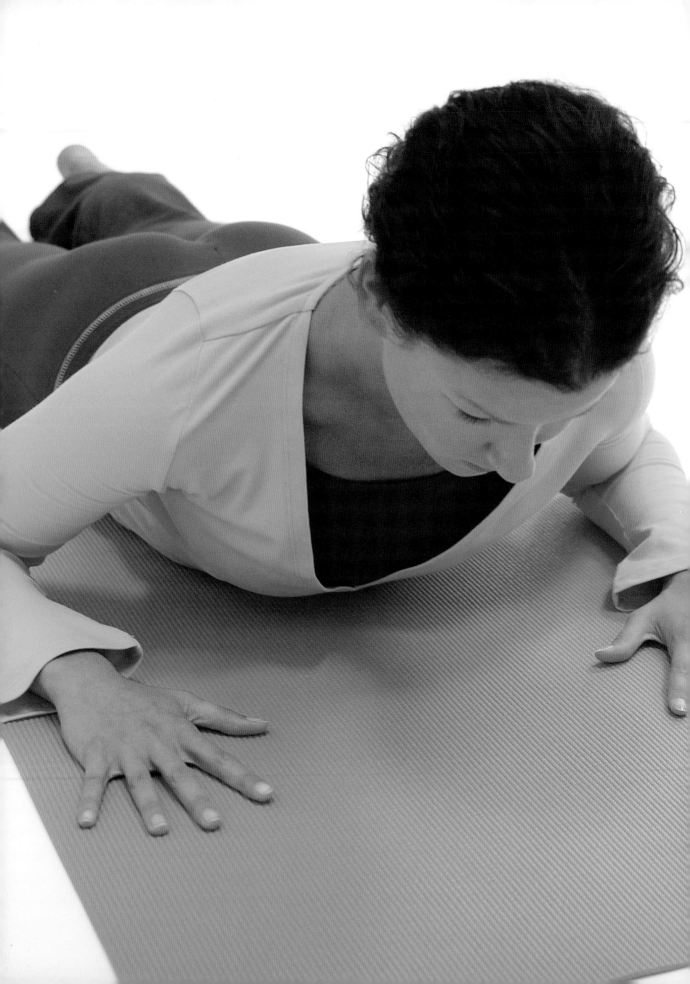

AFTER
THE BIRTH

CHANGES IN YOUR BODY

Congratulations! Your baby is finally here. The next few weeks as a new mum will be both exciting and intense. You will start adjusting your life to cater for your new family member, but you must also make time to look after yourself.

You will now be producing breast milk. Breastfeeding is of course best for your baby and it will help to create a loving bond between the two of you. However, at first it is not always the magical experience you imagined! You may experience nipple soreness and breast discomfort, caused by yet another increase in size as your breasts swell with milk.

Your uterus will take about six weeks before it returns to normal. Soon after the birth you may start to feel it contracting. These contractions are often more intense during breastfeeding.

Within 24 hours of the birth you should be able to resume your pelvic-floor exercises.

If you had a Caesarean birth, it is also important to start exercising your pelvic floor as soon as possible, provided your doctor or midwife has given you the go-ahead. You may find that when you first rise into a standing position, your Caesarean abdominal incision feels odd. The uncomfortable feeling may compel you to bend over and round your back, as you unconsciously try to ease the discomfort in the scar area. Good posture may be hard to maintain at this stage.

Naturally your centre of attention will be on the needs of your baby, but it is easy to neglect your own health. A good recovery for you means a more energetic mum, better able to cope with the demands of your baby.

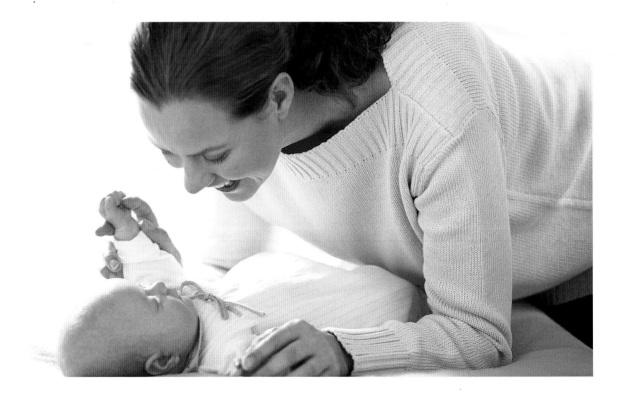

GUIDELINES FOR THE FIRST SIX WEEKS
AFTER VAGINAL BIRTH

- The exercises from birth to six weeks following a vaginal birth are safe for you, subject to your doctor's approval.

- Pelvic-floor exercises may be resumed 24 hours after the birth.

- If you had a perineal tear or episiotomy, you will have had stitches and will be feeling sore. Consult your doctor about scar-tissue management.

- You will find you tire easily, so don't overdo it. Ensure you build up your exercise programme gradually, as many of your physical changes from pregnancy will still be evident.

- Your joints will still be lax and therefore potentially unstable. Keep movements slow and controlled. Avoid over-stretching.

- Avoid exercising too soon after eating a meal.

- Empty your bladder before starting your Pilates session – you will be more comfortable and will not need to interrupt your programme.

- Feed your baby before you exercise to avoid discomfort from heavy, leaking breasts or being interrupted by an upset, hungry baby.

- Pay attention to your technique and how you perform each movement. Quality of movement is more beneficial than quantity.

- Daily walking will help you shed extra pounds, improve your cardiovascular fitness and give you and your baby the psychological benefits of being out in the fresh air.

- If you suffered from carpal tunnel syndrome during pregnancy, it may still be a problem. Use a rolled-up towel under your wrists when doing exercises that put pressure on them. When pushing your baby's buggy, try placing your hands on the sides of the buggy's handles to avoid aggravating the condition.

- Invest in a good-quality sports bra with the maximum amount of support. Look for wide straps to eliminate neck, shoulder and upper back pain. Ensure that your breasts are supported equally, with no cutting or chafing.

- Practise exercises to strengthen your mid-back. Holding, feeding and lifting your baby all conspire against good posture. Following the exercise programmes will give you excellent results.

- Reinforce your posture! Practise standing and walking with poise and sitting well (see pages 14–19). Maintaining good posture now is vital. Poor posture will make you look older and fatter.

- Drink a minimum of eight glasses of water a day, and more if exercising. Adequate hydration is essential if you are breastfeeding. Alcohol and drinking too much coffee will dehydrate you and disturb your sleep patterns.

- Continue to take care when lying and sitting from a standing position and getting up again.

- If something hurts, STOP. This is your body's way of telling you it is not right.

112 AFTER THE BIRTH

GUIDELINES FOR THE FIRST SIX WEEKS AFTER CAESAREAN BIRTH

- Consult your midwife or doctor before you begin any exercising.

- If you had a Caesarean delivery, you must follow the special Caesarean exercise programme (see page 115) to meet your individual needs.

- It is important to start exercising your pelvic floor as soon as you can, provided your doctor or midwife has given you the go-ahead.

- Muscle-wasting must be avoided. With your doctor's approval, begin walking as soon as possible to aid your recovery. Walking will improve your circulation, which can speed the healing process of the incision area.

- Avoid heavy lifting and any strenuous activity for at least six weeks after the birth.

- Avoid doing too much in the early days following your Caesarean. Progress at your own individual pace and only after consultation with your doctor or midwife.

- Your joints will still be lax and therefore potentially unstable. Keep movements slow and controlled. Avoid over-stretching.

- Avoid exercising too soon after eating a meal.

- Empty your bladder before starting your Pilates session – you will be more comfortable and will not need to interrupt your programme.

- Feed your baby before you exercise to avoid discomfort from heavy, leaking breasts or being interrupted by an upset, hungry baby.

- Pay attention to your technique and how you perform each exercise. Quality of movement is more beneficial than quantity.

- If you suffered from carpal tunnel syndrome during pregnancy, it may still be a problem. Use a rolled-up towel under your wrists when you are doing exercises that will put pressure on your wrists. When pushing your baby's buggy, try placing your hands on the sides of the buggy's handles to avoid aggravating the condition.

- Invest in a good-quality sports bra with maximum support. Look out for wide straps that will eliminate neck, shoulder and upper back pain. Ensure that your breasts are supported equally, with no cutting or chafing.

- Practise exercises to strengthen your mid-back. Holding, feeding and lifting your baby all conspire against good posture. Following the exercise programmes will give you excellent results.

- Reinforce your posture! Discomfort around the scar area may cause you to bend over (see 'Taking care of posture' on pages 14–19). Poor posture will make you look older and fatter.

- Drink a minimum of eight glasses of water a day, and more if exercising. Adequate hydration is essential if you are breastfeeding. Alcohol and drinking too much coffee will dehydrate you and disturb your sleep patterns.

- If something hurts, STOP. This is your body's way of telling you it is not right.

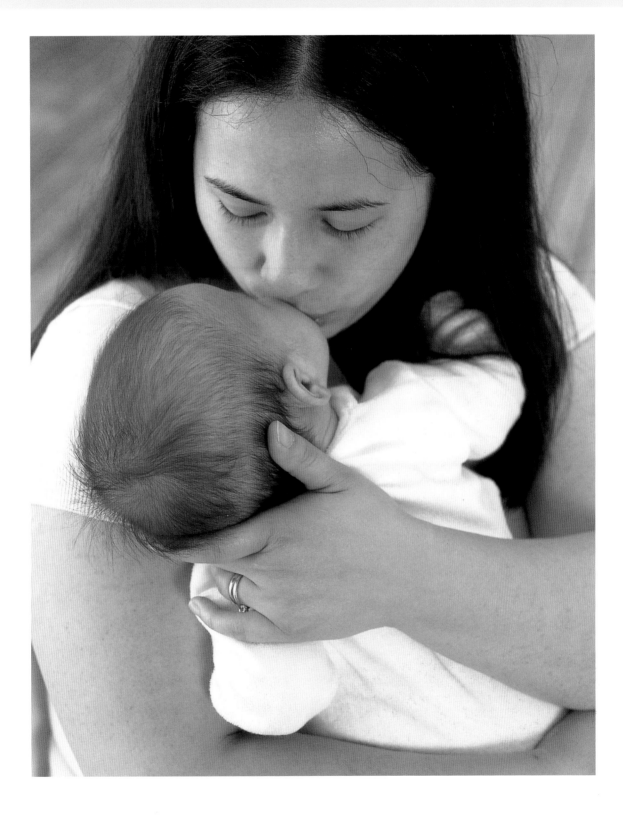

POST-PREGNANCY WORKOUT

By following the essential exercise guidelines for six weeks after the birth and choosing the programme appropriate to the type of birth you had, you will be able to resume safe and effective exercising. These programmes will help you to regain, and improve, your pre-pregnancy figure. The pelvic-floor exercises will give you an excellent start and are easy to do anywhere. You will be eager to lose weight and get back into shape, but do not expect your weight loss to follow a steady downward course. It may see-saw daily, affected by factors such as what you have just eaten, whether you have been exercising, water retention or dehydration. Step on the scales once a week in the morning and before eating.

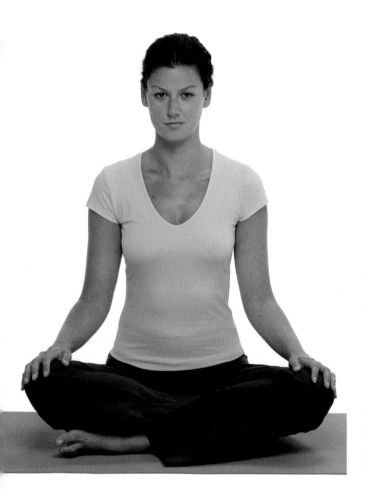

EXERCISES TO STRENGTHEN THE PELVIC FLOOR

Start your pelvic-floor exercises 24 hours after the birth. Using each time you touch water as a memory trigger, practise in sets of five contractions. This not only reinforces what you have practised throughout your pregnancy, but also helps to strengthen the pelvic floor when it needs it most. (You no longer need to practise the Diamond Release, as this was to prepare you for the birth.)

Diamond Lift	page 32
The Big Lift	page 33
Diamond Pulse	page 33

GENTLE EXERCISES FOR SIX WEEKS AFTER VAGINAL BIRTH

When you are comfortable with your workout, you can progress by adding the following exercises to your routine:

GENTLE EXERCISES FOR SIX WEEKS AFTER A CAESAREAN BIRTH

Check with your doctor or midwife before starting these exercises.

Add the following exercises to your workout when you feel less tired or need more of a challenge:

SIX WEEKS AFTER THE BIRTH

Six weeks after your baby's birth you should be feeling ready to resume your normal programme of exercise, provided you had a vaginal delivery with no complications. If you had a Caesarean delivery it is essential that you are cleared by your doctor to resume exercise.

Your body is not necessarily back to its pre-pregnancy state. Your 'six-pack' muscles, the rectus abdominis, have in some cases still not closed after separating to accommodate the baby's growth. While the gap, the diastasis recti (see page 118), remains wider than two fingers, you should not perform Ab Curls (see page 123) or Knee Rolls (see page 120). Check by using the diastasis recti self-test.

Many women experience post-natal depression from all the unsettling hormonal changes that occur during pregnancy. Your new baby's constant demands to be fed, changed and cuddled often lead to fatigue and lack of sleep, which can prompt feelings of depression. You may find it difficult to believe, but exercising can be your saviour! Exercising is a natural mood-enhancer, so keeping your workouts going after the birth is vital, both for your physical and psychological well being. Pilates' tranquil, controlled approach will help you feel calm, strong and in control.

Keep in mind that you are a mum now, so everything you plan to do has to balance with all the other demands on you as a person.

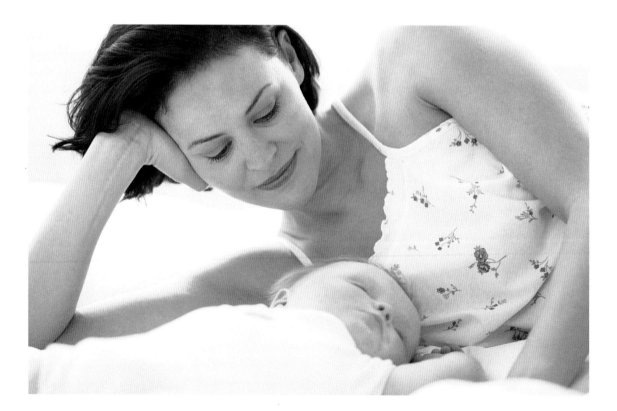

GUIDELINES FROM SIX WEEKS AFTER THE BIRTH

- Approach your exercising slowly and gently, and never hurry. Use the thought processes you have practised throughout your pregnancy to enhance your self-awareness.

- Always breastfeed your baby before you exercise, otherwise your breasts will feel heavy and uncomfortable and you may leak milk. You will also avoid an agitated, hungry baby yelling as you try to exercise calmly!

- Invest in a good-quality sports bra, with maximum support, for your exercise sessions. Look for wide straps to eliminate neck, shoulder and upper back pain. Ensure that your breasts are supported equally, with no cutting or chafing. Note that your nursing bra will not give you the required support when exercising.

- Keep your sessions short so that you do not overtire yourself, which could affect your milk supply.

- Remember that a series of short, calm workouts has the same positive and cumulative effect as one big workout.

- Lying on your stomach is now possible, so you may comfortably resume exercises such as Swimming (see page 56) and The Kite (see page 60).

- Practise your pelvic-floor exercises daily, whenever you touch water. This is such a useful cue because, with all the nappy changing and washing of hands there is no excuse not to do 50 exercises daily.

- Reinforce your posture! Practise standing and walking with poise and sitting well (see pages 16–19). Maintaining good posture now is vital, and poor posture will make you look older and fatter.

- If you feel that your pelvic floor is less sensitive than it was, a good exercise is to place a finger inside your vagina and practise squeezing it. You can also do this squeezing action during intercourse, which is a pleasant way of helping your intimate parts return to normal.

- The hormone relaxin is still present in your body, continuing to keep your muscles and joints lax. Avoid wide ranges of movement, and do not stretch the hamstrings and inner thighs as this will place pressure on the pubis symphysis (see page 12).

- Avoid exercising too soon after eating a meal.

- Empty your bladder before starting your Pilates session – you will be more comfortable and will not need to interrupt your programme.

- Drink a minimum of eight glasses of water a day, and more if exercising. Adequate hydration is essential if you are breastfeeding. Alcohol and drinking too much coffee will dehydrate you and disturb your sleep patterns.

- Set yourself some clearly defined goals. Write them down as monthly targets towards your main goal, and record your activities and progress.

- If you had a Caesarean delivery, the post-pregnancy workouts (see pages 118–125) will specify which exercises you should not be performing.

- If something hurts, STOP. This is your body's way of telling you it is not right.

BACK IN SHAPE EXERCISES

You will now be able to embark on the mini-workout plans (see pages 124–125), which are designed to help you regain your figure, improve your fitness and posture, and make you feel on top of the world. Before you start, there are four wonderful new exercises for you to learn, which you will then find incorporated into the mini-workouts. The new movements will help improve your core stability and will add variety to your exercise sessions.

If you had a Caesarean delivery and your doctor has cleared you to start exercising, you will find there are certain exercises in the mini-workout plans that you should not perform; these are clearly stated as not being suitable for you.

If you still have diastasis recti, you should not perform the Knee Roll (see page 120) or the Ab-Curl (see page 123). You may, however, do the Supported Ab-Curl exercise (see page 122).

You should perform cardiovascular exercise in addition to your mini-workouts, ideally five times a week. Aim for 30 minutes a day, which can be performed in one session, two 15-minute sessions or even three ten-minute sessions each day. Exercise that utilizes the large muscles and strengthens your heart and lungs is beneficial.

Walking is safe and appropriate for all fitness levels, and you can increase the challenge by power-walking and including gradients. Swimming is excellent, easy on your joints and you can take your baby with you too. Even everyday chores such as washing floors and cleaning windows take on a positive aspect, as they too can help you lose extra pregnancy weight.

DIASTASIS RECTI: THE SELF-TEST

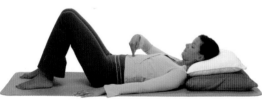

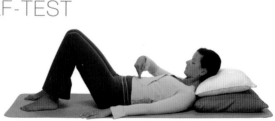

- Lie on your back, with your knees bent and your feet flat on the floor, hip-width apart.

- Place one or two small pillows under your head to ensure that your head and shoulders are higher than your abdomen.

- Rest the fingertips of one hand on your stomach, just above your navel.

- Slowly lift your head and shoulders off the pillows.

- Press firmly with your fingers. If you feel a separation between the two bands of vertical muscle, greater than the width of two fingers (or more than 2 cm/¾ in), then there is separation.

- Check with your doctor or midwife if you are unsure or have any concerns.

This fantastic toning and strengthening exercise works the buttock muscles and improves core strength and stability. During pregnancy you were carrying the weight of your baby in front of you, and this placed extra stress on your buttocks. The Shoulder Bridge strengthens your buttocks and hamstrings, gently lengthening the front thigh muscles. Use a softball for this exercise.

GENTLE HINTS

- Avoid arching your spine, and do not lift your back higher than your shoulder blades.

- Create a diagonal line from shoulders to knees, like a bridge.

- Keep your weight evenly distributed on both feet as you raise your buttocks.

Repetitions: 5–10

1 Lie on your back, with your knees bent and the softball between your knees. Place your feet flat on the floor and hip-width apart. Put your arms by your sides with your palms facing down. Keep your spine in a neutral position. Breathe into the sides and back of your ribcage.

2 Breathe out, pulling your navel in towards your spine, and maintain this contraction throughout. Press your knees against the ball and squeeze your buttocks as you lift them off the floor. Breathe in at the top of the movement, then breathe out as you lengthen back down to the start position. Repeat.

KNEE ROLL

If you have diastasis recti (a gap of 2 cm/¾ in or more in the abdominal muscles, see page 118) or had a Caesarean section, do not perform Knee Rolls. This exercise works the muscles of the waistline. With an emphasis on stability, it will teach you how to safely rotate the spine while lengthening. Holding a rolled-up towel between your knees helps you maintain hip and knee alignment while gently activating your inner thighs. Place a small pillow under your head for comfort.

GENTLE HINTS

- Keep your feet close together throughout this exercise.

- Roll your knees to the side only as far as is comfortable.

Repetitions: 5–10

1 Lie on your back with your knees bent and a rolled-up towel between your knees. Keep your feet together and flat on the mat. Position your arms out to the sides, slightly lower than shoulder level, with the palms facing up. Breathe into the sides and back of your ribcage.

2 Breathe out, pulling your navel in towards your spine and maintaining this contraction throughout. Squeezing the towel, slowly roll your knees to the right, turning your head to the left and turning your left palm face down. Don't let your left shoulder lift off the floor. Breathe in and then, as you breathe out, bring your knees back to the start position. Turn your head back to the centre and face your palm back up. Repeat on the opposite side.

THE SPHINX

Many women complain that they experience lower back pain in the months following the baby's birth. This weakness in the lower back can be exacerbated by all the lifting and holding of your baby, and continues with the habit of always carrying your baby on your hip. This simple yet highly effective exercise will strengthen your lower back muscles, your abdominals and your pelvic floor. Perform this movement slowly and never force it, going only as far as feels comfortable.

Repetitions: 5–10

GENTLE HINTS

- As you lift your head, keep your eye-line aimed at the edge of the exercise mat in front of you.

- Keep your bottom rib in contact with the mat.

- Concentrate on keeping your buttocks and abdominals contracted, to help support the lower back.

1 Lie face down, with your forehead resting on the mat and your feet slightly apart. Place a flat cushion under your forehead for comfort, if you wish. Position your hands beside your head, with your arms bent and your palms facing down. Breathe into the sides and back of your ribcage.

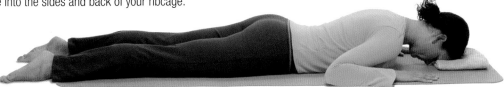

2 Breathe out, lift your pelvic floor and pull your navel in towards your spine. Contract your buttocks, draw your shoulder blades down your back and lift your head and shoulders off the floor. Lengthen the top of your head away from your tailbone. Breathe in and hold for one second, then breathe out as you lengthen back down to the start position. Repeat.

Do not perform this exercise until your doctor has cleared you after your six-week post-natal check. If you have diastasis recti (a gap of 2 cm/^{3}/$_4$ in or more in the abdominal muscles, see page 118), this version of the Ab-Curl is a good one for you. It is not suitable if you had a Caesarean section. The Supported Ab-Curl is an introduction to abdominal curls, known as curl-ups. Performing this exercise slowly helps to close the gap between your abdominal muscles. You will need a towel.

GENTLE HINTS

- Do not lift your shoulders, as this may cause the muscle separation to increase.

- Perform the exercise very slowly and with control.

- As you lift your head, let your eye-line follow a natural path from the ceiling towards your knees.

- If anything feels uncomfortable – STOP.

Repetitions: 5–10

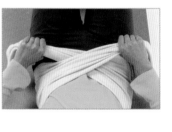

1 Lie on your back, with your knees bent, your feet flat on the floor and hip-width apart. Place a folded towel under your back at waist level, crossing the towel over in front of your stomach. Firmly hold each end of the towel, with your palms facing down. Breathe in, lengthening the back of your neck.

2 Breathe out, slowly pulling your navel in towards your spine. At the same time, gently pull down on the towel so that it tightens across your stomach. Gently raise your head, but keep your shoulders on the mat. Pull the towel firmly across your stomach like a corset, in order to support your abdominals. Breathe in and gently lower to the start position. Repeat.

AB-CURL

Do not perform this exercise until after your six-week post-natal check. This exercise is not suitable if you still have diastasis recti (a gap of 2 cm/$^3/_4$ in or more in the abdominal muscles, see page 118) or if you had a Caesarean section. This popular exercise strengthens your abdominals without allowing the muscles to bulge and pop up. The core-connector techniques practised throughout your pregnancy will now ensure that you target and utilize the correct muscles to help you achieve a toned, flat stomach.

GENTLE HINTS

- Keep your spine in a neutral position throughout, and avoid tucking in your pelvis and clenching your buttocks.

- Do not curl up too high or you will make your abdominals pop up.

- When breathing in, your eye-line moves forward along the ceiling and down towards your knees.

- Maintain a gap the size of an orange between your chin and chest.

Repetitions: 5–10

1 Lie on your back, with your feet flat on the floor and hip-width apart. Place a softball between your knees. Put your hands behind your head without linking your fingers, and keep your elbows open.

2 Breathe in and lengthen the back of your neck. Breathe out, lift your pelvic floor and pull your navel in towards your spine. Simultaneously stabilize your shoulder blades and, maintaining length in your neck, curl your head and shoulders off the mat. Now breathe in, holding your contracted abdominals flat. Breathe out as you roll your upper body down to the mat. Repeat.

MINI-WORKOUTS

These ten-minute mini-workouts are ideal for the busy mum when time is short. These four workouts will cover all your fitness needs, and you will find a recommended frequency with each workout. However, if you feel the need, there is nothing to stop you doing two of these workouts in one day, performing one in the morning and another in the afternoon. Just don't overdo it! Always perform your warm-up exercises before commencing a workout.

AT-A-GLANCE WARM-UP

The warm-up exercises come from the Pilates Basics section (see pages 24–41). Perform them in the order listed below:

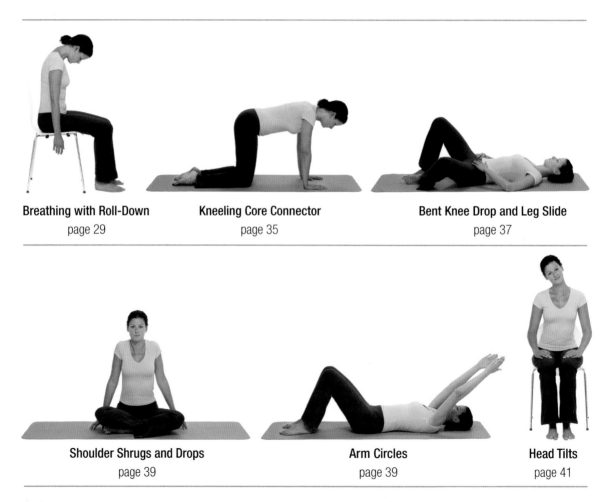

Breathing with Roll-Down
page 29

Kneeling Core Connector
page 35

Bent Knee Drop and Leg Slide
page 37

Shoulder Shrugs and Drops
page 39

Arm Circles
page 39

Head Tilts
page 41

You are now warmed up and ready to begin any of the Mini-Workouts on the opposite page.
Study the plan of your choice, then learn the exercises.

POSTURE PLUS

Perform three times a week:

Seated Row	page 72
Chest Opener	page 81
Shoulder Bridge	page 119
Kneeling Core Connector & Core Connector with Ball	page 35
Ab-Curl* or Supported Ab-Curl**	pages 122/123
Knee Rolls*	page 120
The Sphinx	page 121
Kneeling Spine Release	page 63

UPPER BODY TONER

Perform twice a week:

Wall Press	page 48
Seated Row	page 72
Kneeling Spine Release	page 63
Overhead Reach	page 49
Barn Doors	page 54
Hammer Curl	page 99
Triceps Toner	page 53
Posture Prompter	page 74

LOWER BACK CARE

Perform three times a week:

Spine Wave	page 77
Kneeling Core Connector & Core Connector with Ball	page 35
Ab-Curl* or Supported Ab-Curl**	pages 122/123
Shoulder Bridge	page 119
The Sphinx	page 121
The Cat	page 82
Swimming (legs only)	page 56
Kneeling Spine Release	page 63

LOWER BODY TONER

Perform twice a week:

Tip & Dip	page 95
Shoulder Bridge	page 119
Ball Squeezer	page 61
Round-the-Clock	page 84
Superwoman (legs only)	page 78
Kneeling Spine Release	page 63
Wall Squat	page 102
Calf Stretch	page 76

* not suitable if you have diastasis recti or had a Caesarean delivery ** not suitable if you had a Caesarean delivery

ACKNOWLEDGEMENTS

AUTHOR ACKNOWLEDGEMENTS

A big thank you goes to Michael Harrison for his help and encouragement in the writing of this book. My appreciation goes to my clients, who continue to inspire me with their enthusiasm for my teaching methods and for the results they achieve. Thank you to the team at Hamlyn for their friendly guidance and help, and to Mike Prior for his excellent photography. Special mention goes to my family for their constant patience and support.

PUBLISHER ACKNOWLEDGEMENTS

Executive Editor Jane McIntosh
Editor Charlotte Macey
Executive Art Editor Karen Sawyer
Designer Janis Utton
Illustrator Trevor Bounford
Photographer Mike Prior
Production Manager Ian Paton
Picture Researcher Sophie Delpech

Thank you to Agoy for the loan of yoga mats for photography
www.agoy.com

Special photography
©Octopus Publishing Group Limited/Mike Prior.

Other photography
DigitalVision 66, 110, 116. Octopus Publishing Group Limited/Adrian Pope 113; /Russell Sadur 45. PhotoDisc 9, 88.